USER'S GUIDE FOR

STRUCTURED CLINICAL INTERV
FOR DSM-IV AXIS II PERSONALITY DI

SCID-II

Michael B. First, M.D.
Miriam Gibbon, M.S.W.
Robert L. Spitzer, M.D.
Janet B. W. Williams, D.S.W.

Biometrics Research Department
New York State Psychiatric Institute
Department of Psychiatry
Columbia University
New York, New York

Lorna Smith Benjamin, Ph.D.

Department of Psychology
University of Utah
Salt Lake City, Utah

Note: The authors have worked to ensure that all information in this book is accurate at the time of publication and consistent with general psychiatric and medical standards. As medical research and practice continue to advance, however, therapeutic standards may change. Moreover, specific situations may require a specific therapeutic response not included in this book. For these reasons, and because human and mechanical errors sometimes occur, we recommend that readers follow the advice of physicians and therapists directly involved in their care or the care of a member of their family.

Manufactured in the United States of America on acid-free paper
09 08 4 3

American Psychiatric Publishing, Inc.
1000 Wilson Boulevard, Arlington, VA 22209-3901

ISBN 0-88048-810-7

For citation: First MB, Gibbon M, Spitzer RL, Williams JBW, Benjamin LS: User's Guide for the Structured Clinical Interview for DSM-IV Axis II Personality Disorders (SCID-II). Washington, DC, American Psychiatric Press, 1997.

Available From American Psychiatric Press:

Structured Clinical Interview for DSM-IV Axis II Personality Disorders (SCID-II)

- User's Guide (order #8810)

  The ***User's Guide*** *contains detailed instructions for administering the SCID-II. It contains sections describing the rationale and structure of the SCID-II and a detailed item-by-item commentary. A sample case is also included to help clinicians learn to use the SCID-II.*

- Packet of five Interviews and five Questionnaires (order #8811)

  The single-use ***Interview*** *contains the interview questions and provides space for recording diagnostic decisions and descriptive information. At the conclusion of the Interview, the clinician completes the Summary Scoresheet and computes a dimensional score for each personality disorder. The single-use* ***Personality Questionnaire*** *to be completed by the patient can be used as a screening tool to shorten the Interview. It is bound separately, but sold only with the Interview booklet.*

- SET of User's Guide + Packet of five Interviews & five Questionnaires (order #8812)

Author's Note: Some of the information describing the SCID-II was adapted in part from First MB, Spitzer RL, Gibbon M, Williams JBW: "The Structured Clinical Interview for DSM-III-R Personality Disorders (SCID-II), Part I: Description." *Journal of Personality Disorders* 9:2 (June 1995).

ACKNOWLEDGMENTS

The development of the SCID was supported in part by NIMH Contract #278-83-007(DB) and NIMH Grant #1 R01 MH40511.

Drafts of the DSM-IV SCID-II were made available to some experienced SCIDers, who provided extremely helpful suggestions: Tom Bartlett, Lynn Gladis, Hillary Glick, and Suzanne Sunday.

CONTENTS

1. Introduction

The Structured Clinical Interview for DSM-IV Axis II Personality Disorders (SCID-II) is a semistructured diagnostic interview for assessing the 10 DSM-IV (American Psychiatric Association 1994) Axis II personality disorders, as well as Depressive Personality Disorder and Passive-Aggressive Personality Disorder (included in DSM-IV's Appendix B, "Criteria Sets and Axes Provided for Further Study"). SCID-II can be used to make Axis II diagnoses, either categorically (present or absent) or dimensionally (by noting the number of personality disorder criteria for each diagnosis that are coded "3").

The SCID-II can be used in both research and clinical settings. SCID-II has been used in three different types of studies. Some studies have used SCID-II to characterize the profile of personality disorders for a sample either in a particular setting or with particular characteristics (e.g., patients with panic disorder) (Brooks et al. 1991; Friedman et al. 1987; Green and Curtis 1988; Lofgren et al. 1991). Other studies have used SCID-II to select individuals from a general setting who have a particular diagnosis (Schotte et al. 1991a, 1991b). Finally, some studies have used SCID-II for comparison with other assessment methods for personality disorders (O'Boyle & Self 1990; Renneberg et al. 1992).

In clinical settings, the SCID-II can be used in at least three ways. In the first way, the clinician does his or her usual clinical interview and then uses a portion of the SCID-II to confirm and document one or more suspected DSM-IV Personality Disorder diagnoses. For example, hearing that the patient has a history of unstable relationships with dramatic endings, the clinician may choose to use the sections of the SCID-II covering the Cluster B Personality Disorders (i.e., Antisocial, Borderline, Histrionic, and Narcissistic Personality Disorders). In this instance, the SCID-II provides the clinician not only with the actual DSM-IV criteria for these disorders, but also with the SCID-II questions that are efficient and effective ways of eliciting the information necessary to judge the diagnostic criteria. In the second way, the SCID-II (and, optionally, the SCID-II Personality Questionnaire) are administered as an Axis II intake procedure. Finally, the SCID-II can be helpful in improving the interview skills of students in the mental health professions. The SCID-II can provide them with a repertoire of useful questions to elicit information that will be the basis for making judgments about the diagnostic criteria. Through repeated administrations of the SCID-II, students become familiar with the DSM-IV criteria for Personality Disorders and at the same time incorporate useful questions into their interviewing repertoire.

Throughout this User's Guide, we have opted to use the terms "interviewer" and "subject" to refer to the administrator of the SCID-II and the person being evaluated, respectively. When used in clinical settings, please mentally substitute the words "clinician" and "patient"/"client" when reading through this manual.

2. History

The origins of SCID-II can be traced to the early stages of the Structured Clinical Interview for DSM-III (SCID), when a personality disorders module developed by Dr. Jeffrey Jonas of McLean Hospital was included in the 1984 version of SCID. In 1985, the SCID personality disorders module was reformulated into a separate, stand-alone instrument for a number of reasons, including the length of the module, burgeoning research interest in personality disorders, and the special assessment requirements for personality features. In 1986, SCID-II was updated for DSM-III-R and a new strategy, with a screening personality questionnaire, was incorporated. After field trials establishing the reliability of SCID-II were completed (First et al. 1995), a final version of SCID-II for DSM-III-R personality disorders was published by American Psychiatric Press, Inc., in 1990 as a component of the SCID. After the publication of DSM-IV in 1994, work was begun on revising SCID-II for DSM-IV. With the help of

Dr. Lorna Benjamin, many of the SCID-II questions were reworded to make them more reflective of the subject's inner experience. This final free-standing version of SCID-II for DSM-IV was published in 1997 by American Psychiatric Press, Inc., with an accompanying computerized version published by Multi-Health Systems of Toronto, Canada (see Section 7: Data Processing for more information).

3. SCID-II Features

3.1 Coverage of SCID-II

SCID-II covers all 10 of the DSM-IV personality disorders, as well as Personality Disorder Not Otherwise Specified, Passive-Aggressive Personality Disorder, and Depressive Personality Disorder—which are included in Appendix B of DSM-IV—also can be diagnosed with SCID-II. Ordinarily, the entire SCID-II is administered; however, it is also possible to administer only those sections relating to personality disorders that are of particular interest to the clinician or researcher.

3.2 Basic Structure

The basic structure of SCID-II is similar to that of the SCID for Axis I disorders. Modeled on the clinical interview, the instrument begins with a brief overview that characterizes the subject's usual behavior and relationships and provides information about the subject's capacity for self-reflection. The SCID-II Overview starts with the statement, "Now I am going to ask you some questions about the kind of person you are—that is, how you generally have felt or behaved." This statement is followed by a number of open-ended questions intended to assess general personality characteristics, such as, "How would you describe yourself as a person?" "What kinds of things have you done that other people might have found annoying?" "If you could change your personality in some ways, how would you want to be different?"

Next, each of the 10 specific personality disorders and 2 appendix categories are considered in turn: Avoidant Personality Disorder, Dependent Personality Disorder, Obsessive-Compulsive Personality Disorder, Passive-Aggressive Personality Disorder, Depressive Personality Disorder, Paranoid Personality Disorder, Schizotypal Personality Disorder, Schizoid Personality Disorder, Histrionic Personality Disorder, Narcissistic Personality Disorder, Borderline Personality Disorder, and Antisocial Personality Disorder. The ordering of the personality disorders in SCID-II differs from that of the DSM-IV classification in order to facilitate rapport with the subject by not beginning with the "odd" A cluster (paranoid, schizoid, schizotypal). Finally, a diagnosis of Personality Disorder Not Otherwise Specified can be given to indicate cases in which personality disorder features are present that do not meet the full criteria for any specific disorder, yet cause significant impairment in functioning.

Like the SCID for Axis I disorders, SCID-II has three columns: the left-hand column contains the interview questions; the center column lists the DSM-IV diagnostic criteria; and the right-hand column is for making the item ratings.

Each personality disorder criterion is rated as either "?," "1," "2," or "3."

? = Inadequate information to code the criterion as either 1, 2, or 3

For example, a subject denies being interpersonally exploitative, but the referral notes state "rule out Narcissistic Personality Disorder."

When subsequent information makes it possible to recode the criterion, the "?" should be crossed out and a circle made around the correct code. In the above example, the Narcissistic Personality Disorder item is recoded "3" after speaking with family members and prior therapists who are able to describe a pattern of exploitative behavior.

1 = Absent or False

Absent. The symptom described in the criterion is clearly absent (e.g., no evidence of identity disturbance).

False. The criterion statement is clearly false (e.g., only one of five required symptoms present).

2 = Subthreshold

The threshold for the criterion is almost, but not quite, met (e.g., interpersonal difficulties occur with current boyfriend but no past boyfriends; trait is present but not severe enough to cause impairment or distress).

3 = Threshold or True

Threshold. The threshold for the criterion is just met (e.g., subject acknowledges trait and describes one convincing example) or is more than met (e.g., subject reports a number of convincing examples in multiple contexts). See section 4.2 for a more detailed discussion of the criteria for rating a "3."

True. The criterion statement is true (e.g., four or more obsessive-compulsive personality disorder items are coded "3").

In most cases, there is one numbered SCID-II interview question for each personality disorder criterion. Some criteria, particularly those that may be more difficult to assess in an interview format (e.g., identity disturbance in Borderline Personality Disorder), have several numbered SCID-II questions that attempt to address different aspects of the criterion. In such cases, the interviewer should ask as many of these numbered questions as needed to gather enough evidence to determine whether the item should be rated a "3." For example, three numbered questions are provided for the assessment of the first criterion for Schizotypal Personality Disorder ("ideas of reference"). If the patient provides enough convincing examples of referential thinking in response to the first question (i.e., "When you are out in public and see people talking, do you often feel that they are talking about you?"), there is no need to explore the other two numbered questions. However, if the answer to the first numbered question is negative (or the patient cannot provide convincing examples), the other numbered questions must be explored as alternatives. The numbered questions are written in such a way as to be overly sensitive (i.e., many subjects will answer "yes" to the numbered questions without truly having the personality features encapsulated in the criterion). For this reason, follow-up questions (which are not numbered) need to be asked only if the subject's response to the numbered question is positive. The follow-up questions serve to elicit corroborating evidence from the subject to establish that the criterion item is present at the threshold level. Often, the follow-up question is a request for examples in the subject's own words. If, after asking the provided follow-up question, the interviewer feels that the subject has not provided enough information to make a definitive rating, the interviewer is encouraged to ad lib as many additional questions as needed.

3.3 SCID-II Scoresheet

The presence of each personality disorder is determined as the interview progresses. At the conclusion of the interview, the interviewer completes the Summary Scoresheet, on which a dimensional score is computed for each personality disorder by summing the number of items rated as positive. For each disorder, a box indicates the DSM-IV categorical threshold (i.e., the number of items required to make the diagnosis). In the common situation in which the criteria for more than one personality disorder are met, the interviewer is instructed to indicate the "principal Axis II diagnosis" (i.e., the personality disorder that is, or should be, the main focus of clinical attention) by recording the two-digit code (located to the left of each diagnosis on the scoresheet) on the bottom of the scoresheet.

3.4 Sources of Information

The subject of the interview frequently is the sole source of information; however, the interviewer should use any sources available when making the ratings, including information from a current or previous therapist or from family members. Ancillary information may be especially important in the evaluation of personality disorders because of a tendency for subjects to underreport personality pathology. Although not specifically designed for this purpose, SCID-II may be administered to an informant about the subject. In cases in which contradictory information is elicited, the interviewer must use his or her clinical judgment in determining whether the informant or the subject is giving the more valid account.

4. Administering SCID-II

4.1 Axis I Pre-evaluation

Ordinarily, SCID-II is administered following an Axis I SCID evaluation, which may have been given on a previous occasion. If an Axis I SCID evaluation has not been conducted, SCID-II should be administered following an unstructured clinical interview that reviews the major Axis I disorders. This procedure serves two purposes. The first purpose is to help identify any circumscribed periods during which an Axis I disorder, such as an episode of Major Depressive Disorder, may have occurred. Such an episode may have been associated with time-limited behaviors that should not be confused with long-term personality functioning. The second purpose is to obtain background information that is useful in the evaluation of the responses to SCID-II questions.

4.2 Criteria for a Rating of "3"

As with the SCID for Axis I disorders, the ratings are of items, not of answers to questions. Frequently a subject will answer "yes" to a question, but the interviewer's clinical judgment (after further inquiry) will be that the item should be coded "1" or "2." A rating of "3" is warranted only if the subject has provided a convincing elaboration or example, or if there is clear evidence from behavior during the interview or from other sources that the item meets the threshold requirements for a "3" rating. To facilitate the differentiation of a rating of subthreshold from a rating of threshold, each item includes a specific guideline for making a "3" rating.

Determining whether a particular item should be rated "3" can be quite challenging because of the inherently unclear boundary between a personality disorder item and a "normal" personality trait. In an attempt to clarify the characteristics of a personality disorder, DSM-IV includes a set of general diagnostic criteria (p. 633). Each of these criteria should be considered when determining whether a particular item warrants a rating of "3":

A. An enduring pattern of inner experience and behavior that deviates markedly from the expectations of the individual's culture. All personality traits occur on a continuum. This criterion highlights the fact that, by definition, a personality disorder item must be at the extreme end of that continuum for it to warrant a rating of "3." For example, some degree of social anxiety is present in nearly everyone; however, the item "excessive social anxiety" under Schizotypal Personality Disorder should be coded "3" only if the subject describes examples of social anxiety that clearly are extreme. This criterion also underscores the cultural relativism of the concept of personality disorder. For example, what may seem histrionic in a culture that values restraint may fall well within the cultural norm in a culture that values spontaneity. Thus, it is critically important for the interviewer to be familiar with what is considered to be the "norm" for a particular person's culture. In situations in which the interviewer is not familiar with the culture of the subject being evaluated, it may be helpful (or even necessary) to consult with others who share the subject's cultural reference points before making assumptions about the presence of a personality disorder.

These follow-up questions may be helpful in determining whether a behavior is at the extreme end of the continuum:

- What is that like?
- Give me the most extreme example.
- Do you think you are more this way than most people you know?

B. The enduring pattern is inflexible and pervasive across a broad range of personal and social situations. To justify a rating of "3," there must be evidence that the behavior, cognition, or affect is both inflexible and pervasive. The inflexible nature of a personality trait would lead the individual being evaluated to express this trait consistently across most situations. Therefore, the interviewer should look for evidence that the trait has a pervasive impact on all (or most) areas of personality functioning and is not restricted to a single interpersonal relationship, situation, or role. If the behavior, cognition, or affect has occurred only with one person but not with most others (e.g., with a particular boss but not with all supervisors), it is more likely to represent a relational problem or an adjustment disorder than a personality trait. These follow-up questions may be helpful:

- Does this happen in a lot of different situations?
- Does this happen with a lot of different people?

C. The enduring pattern leads to clinically significant distress or impairment in social, occupational, or other important areas of functioning. Impairment in personality functioning also occurs on a continuum. Only when a personality trait is maladaptive and thus causes significant functional impairment or subjective distress does it warrant a rating of "3." The interviewer should ask questions to determine the negative impact of the trait on the subject's social interactions; the subject's ability to form and maintain close relationships; and the subject's ability to function effectively at work, school, or home.

Because personality traits are commonly egosyntonic (i.e., they involve characteristics that the person accepts as an integral part of the self), the person being evaluated may deny that the trait has any negative impact on his or her functioning. For example, individuals with Obsessive-Compulsive Personality Disorder may consider their perfectionism and incessant devotion to work a cherished quality and an indication of scrupulousness, moral superiority, and dedication. It is important to recognize that subjective distress or a direct acknowledgment of impairment is *not* necessary for a rating of "3." If, in the interviewer's clinical opinion, the trait is having a significantly negative impact on the person's level of functioning, the item can still be rated "3." For example, if a person with no friends who has not been able to advance in his career because of social avoidance rationalizes that he prefers being alone and working in a low-level job, this would warrant a "3" rating on item 1 for Avoidant Personality Disorder.

In assessing impairment or distress, these follow-up questions may be helpful:

- What problems does this cause for you?
- Does it bother other people?

D. The pattern is stable and of long duration, and its onset can be traced back at least to adolescence or early adulthood. Personality traits do not refer to time-limited and discrete episodes of illness. Rather, maladaptive personality traits are, by definition, chronic patterns with an early and insidious onset evident by late adolescence or early adulthood. For the purposes of SCID-II, the concept of "long duration" is operationalized so that a rating of "3" means that the characteristic has been frequently present over a period of at least the last 5 years. (The only exceptions are certain extreme items, such as suicidal behavior, that are diagnostically significant even when they occur relatively infrequently.) Furthermore, there must be some evidence of the trait going back as far as the subject's late teens or early twenties. These follow-up questions may be helpful:

- Have you been this way for a long time?
- How often does this happen?
- When can you first remember [feeling/acting] this way?

E. The enduring pattern is not better accounted for as a manifestation or consequence of another mental disorder. The evaluation of personality disorders in the presence of Axis I conditions often is quite difficult. A subject's current behavior may reflect the presence of an episodic mood or anxiety disorder as opposed to a stable personality disposition. To tease out Axis I versus Axis II relationships, the interviewer must confirm that the trait has been present and long-standing prior to and independent of the Axis I condition. For this reason, the SCID-II Overview has the following statement:

> IF A CIRCUMSCRIBED OR EPISODIC AXIS I DISORDER HAS BEEN PRESENT: I know that there have been times when you have been [AXIS I SYMPTOMS]. I am not talking about those times; you should try to think of how you *usually* are when you are not [AXIS I SYMPTOMS]. Do you have any questions about this?

Furthermore, when determining whether an item should be rated "3" in the presence of an Axis I disorder, it may be helpful to ask the following question: Are you generally this way even when you are not [AXIS I SYMPTOM (e.g., depressed)]? In cases in which the Axis I condition itself has been long-standing and chronic, trying to determine whether the behavior is part of the Axis I disorder or better considered to be a personality trait may be impossible (and ultimately meaningless). In such situations, it probably makes the most sense not to attribute the trait to the Axis I condition and to make a rating of "3."

F. The enduring pattern is not due to the direct physiological effects of a substance (e.g., a drug of abuse, medication, toxin exposure) or a general medical condition (e.g., head trauma). The relationship between some personality disorders (particularly Borderline and Antisocial Personality Disorders) and substance use can be difficult to evaluate. In some people, substance use may be indicative of the impulsivity that is characteristic of these personality disorders or a form of self-medication to regulate the dysphoric mood states that may be associated with them. In others, the behaviors that characterize the "personality disorder" may in fact be secondary to the drug-taking either by direct physiological effect (e.g., the substance causes affective lability) or the fact that obtaining the funds for illegal substances often entails antisocial behavior. In such situations, a careful evaluation comparing the onset of the personality traits and the pattern of substance use may be helpful in assessing their relationship.

The second half of this criterion refers to the differential diagnosis between a personality disorder and personality change due to a general medical condition. Although a number of general medical conditions can result in personality changes, in practice this differential is rarely a problem because of the difference in characteristic age and mode of onset between personality disorder and personality change. In personality disorders, the onset is early (i.e., by age 18) and usually gradual and is not related to a general medical condition. In personality change, the onset can be at any age and must be a direct result of the effects of a general medical condition on the central nervous system. The situation in which this differential may be most difficult to assess is when the "change" occurs in childhood and is not conclusively related to the general medical condition. For example, it may be difficult to evaluate whether antisocial behavior in a child who had pre-existing head trauma is due to the head injury or whether the injury is incidental.

A final caveat: It is important to keep in mind that interviewers have their own enduring styles of personality functioning that may color their perceptions and judgments of the personality functioning of others. For example, an interviewer with obsessive-compulsive traits may have difficulty appreciating the pathological nature of such traits when these are present in others; the same interviewer may be excessively judgmental in evaluating subjects with histrionic features. Social, cultural, and gender biases can further complicate the assessment. For example, interviewers from cultures that place a high value on controlled and compulsive behavior are more likely to see as pathologically histrionic the more spontaneous behavior sanctioned by other cultures, and vice versa. Furthermore, interviewers (whether male or female) may at times be influenced by their stereotypes about "normal" masculine and feminine behavior. Therefore, the interviewer must be aware of possible effects of his or her own biases when determining whether a particular behavior, affect, or cognition is "pathological" and deserving of a rating of "3."

In summary: Remember the three "P"s: A rating of "3" requires that the characteristic described in the item be *pathological* (i.e., outside the range of normal variation), *persistent* (i.e., frequently present over a period of at least the last 5 years with onset by early adulthood), and *pervasive* (i.e., apparent in a variety of contexts, such as at work and at home, or, in the case of items concerning interpersonal relations, in several different relationships).

4.3 Use of SCID-II With SCID-II Personality Questionnaire

A feature unique to SCID-II is the availability of a self-report personality questionnaire as a screening tool to shorten the time required for the clinician to administer the instrument. After the subject fills out the Personality Questionnaire (which usually takes 20 minutes), the clinician simply circles the numbers to the left of the SCID-II items that correspond to items answered "yes" on the questionnaire. When SCID-II is administered, the interviewer need only inquire about the items screened positive on the questionnaire. The assumption is that a subject who responds with a "no" on the questionnaire item would also have answered "no" to the same question had it been read aloud by the interviewer. In either instance, no follow-up questions are appropriate because it is not reasonable to ask the subject to provide examples of a behavior that is not present. The justification for accepting a "no" response on the questionnaire is that a subject who is unwilling to acknowledge a symptom sitting by himself or herself with pencil and paper is unlikely to acknowledge the same symptom when asked by an interviewer.

The Personality Questionnaire requires an eighth grade or higher reading level (as determined by the Flesch-Kincaid formula). Each of the 119 questions on the questionnaire corresponds to an initial interview question in SCID-II (identified by numbers in the left-hand column of both instruments). For example, question 91 on the Personality Questionnaire is, "Do your relationships with people you really care about have lots of extreme ups and downs?" This corresponds to the initial SCID-II interview question (91) for the second criterion in Borderline Personality Disorder. In most cases, the items on the Personality Questionnaire set a threshold for a positive response that is considerably lower than that of the corresponding diagnostic criterion in SCID-II. For example, question 66 on the Personality Questionnaire asks, "Do you like to be the center of attention?" Many individuals will circle "Yes" on the questionnaire, but further questioning during the SCID-II interview may lead the interviewer to conclude that the criterion "Is uncomfortable in situations in which he or she is not the center of attention" will not be met. In other words, the Personality Questionnaire acts as a screening device with intentionally high rates of false positives. It also should produce few false negatives because the interviewer is encouraged to explore items for which there is any evidence during the interview regardless of the subject's response on the questionnaire (e.g., for a subject who acts suspicious during the interview, the interviewer should ask the subject all questions relevant to paranoid ideation, even if answered "no" on the Personality Questionnaire). Because of the intended high false-positive rates, we do not recommend using the Personality Questionnaire as a stand-alone instrument for any purpose other than as a rough screening device.

As previously noted, the interviewer should circle the numbers to the left of the questions on SCID-II that correspond to the items answered "yes" on the Personality Questionnaire. If a Personality Questionnaire item is not answered at all (i.e., neither "yes" nor "no" is circled), then the SCID-II number should be circled and a question mark written on the left. Once all "yes" and unanswered questions are noted on the left-hand side of SCID-II, the interviewer should proceed with SCID-II as follows:

1. For all items with a circled number (i.e., "yes" answer on questionnaire), the interviewer reads the SCID-II question, omitting the italicized text in brackets.

2. For all items without a circled number (i.e., "no" answer on questionnaire), no question is read and the criterion is rated "1." (Note: the interviewer should do this only if confident that this is a true negative—see below for two exceptions.)

3. For all items with a circled number and a question mark (i.e., neither "yes" nor "no" answer on questionnaire), the interviewer reads the SCID-II question using the italicized text and leaving out the initial phrase.

To illustrate this procedure, look at the numbered question corresponding to criterion 1 of Avoidant Personality Disorder: "You've said that you have *[Have you]* avoided jobs or tasks that involved having to deal with a lot of people." If the person being evaluated circled "yes" on question 1 on the Personality Questionnaire, the interviewer would read the question: "You've said that you have avoided jobs or tasks that involved having to deal with a lot of people." If the question was answered "no," no question would be asked and criterion 1 would be rated "1." If neither "yes" nor "no" was circled (e.g., the subject did not understand the question, was unsure of his or her answer, or was too embarrassed to answer), the interviewer would read the question using only the italicized text, leaving out the initial part: "Have you avoided jobs or tasks that involved having to deal with a lot of people?"

Some of the SCID-II items have more than one corresponding Personality Questionnaire question. In such cases, the criterion should be explored if any of the Personality Questionnaire questions have been answered "yes" or left unanswered. In these instances, it is often helpful to re-ask a question that was answered "no." For example, the first item for Narcissistic Personality Disorder ("grandiose sense of self-importance") has two corresponding questions on the Personality Questionnaire (73 and 74). If question 73 was answered "no" and question 74 was answered "yes," criterion 1 should be explored further by asking the subject for examples. If there is still not enough information to decide whether to rate the item "3," the interviewer should re-ask question 73 using the italicized text (even though it was answered "no") to be absolutely sure that it is a true negative.

Using the Personality Questionnaire saves interview time because, in general, items answered "no" on the questionnaire are skipped during the course of the SCID-II interview. However, there are two circumstances in which items that are answered "no" on the questionnaire should be further explored in the SCID-II interview:

- *When there is a clinical basis to suspect that the item is true.* For example, even if a subject has denied all of the items for Narcissistic Personality Disorder on the questionnaire, if the subject presents himself during the interview in a grandiose manner or acts in an entitled manner, the interviewer should explore all of the items for this disorder.
- *When the number of SCID-II items coded "3" is within one item of the diagnostic threshold for a particular disorder.* For example, if three items for Avoidant Personality Disorder are coded "3" (one fewer than the four required), the remaining items should be probed during the SCID-II interview even if they were denied on the questionnaire.

Users who are interested in noting personality traits even when they are insufficient in number to qualify for a personality disorder diagnosis should probe all items coded "yes" on the questionnaire. Those interested only in whether the full criteria are met for the disorders may choose not to probe questionnaire items answered "yes" for disorders for which the number of "yes" items is well below the threshold for the disorder and there is no clinical evidence suggesting that the disorder is present. For example, if "yes" is circled for only two questionnaire items corresponding to the Avoidant Personality Disorder criteria, and there is no clinical evidence in the interview suggesting this disorder, the entire section may be skipped because a minimum of four items is required to make the diagnosis.

4.4 Use of SCID-II Without SCID-II Personality Questionnaire

SCID-II may be administered without the Personality Questionnaire. This may be especially desirable in situations in which the interviewer wishes to focus on a limited number of disorders. When SCID-II is used without the questionnaire, all of the questions should be asked using the italicized phrases in brackets and omitting the initial words preceding the brackets (usually "You've said that. . ."). For example, question 16 (for criterion 1 for Obsessive-Compulsive Personality Disorder) is given in the form, "You've said that you are *[Are you]* the kind of person who focuses on details, order, and organization or likes to make lists and schedules." This would be rephrased as: "Are you the kind of person who focuses on details, order, and organization or likes to make lists and schedules?"

5. SCID-II Item-by-Item Commentary

The next section contains commentaries for each individual personality disorder item. Please refer to this section for help in interpreting the meaning of the criterion and for help in distinguishing the item from similar items in other disorders.

5.1 Avoidant Personality Disorder

(1) avoids occupational activities that involve significant interpersonal contact because of fears of criticism, disapproval, or rejection

> *Interviewer's Questions:* You've said that you have *[Have you]* avoided jobs or tasks that involved having to deal with a lot of people. Give me some examples. What was the reason that you avoided these [LIST JOBS OR TASKS]? (Have you ever refused a promotion because it would involve dealing with more people than you would be comfortable with?)

Commentary: Because of a fear of rejection, or of saying or doing the wrong thing, people with Avoidant Personality Disorder typically avoid jobs or school activities that put them in contact with other people (e.g., "front-desk" assignments or group projects). They prefer to work by themselves and may refuse promotions because the new position would make them more visible—and therefore vulnerable to criticism or humiliation by others.

(2) is unwilling to get involved with people unless certain of being liked

> *Interviewer's Questions:* You've said that *[Do]* you avoid getting involved with people unless you are certain they will like you. If you don't know whether someone likes you, would you ever make the first move?

Commentary: Many people are hesitant to initiate a social interaction because of a fear of being rejected. People with this disorder tend to watch from the sidelines until they are certain they will be accepted. This differs from the next item, which involves putting limits on the intimacy of a close relationship.

(3) shows restraint within intimate relationships because of the fear of being shamed or ridiculed

Interviewer's Questions: You've said that *[Do]* you find it hard to be "open" even with people you are close to. Why is this? (Are you afraid of being made fun of or embarrassed?)

Commentary: Although people with this disorder are able to establish intimate relationships when there is assurance of uncritical acceptance, they have difficulty talking about themselves and withhold intimate feelings for fear of being exposed, ridiculed, or shamed.

(4) is preoccupied with being criticized or rejected in social situations

Interviewer's Questions: You've said that *[Do]* you often worry about being criticized or rejected in social situations. Give me some examples. Do you spend a lot of time worrying about this?

Commentary: People with Avoidant Personality Disorder or Narcissistic Personality Disorder may be hypersensitive to criticism, reacting to even minor criticisms with feelings of hurt or embarrassment. Individuals with Narcissistic Personality Disorder do not expect to be criticized and are surprised, indignant, and outraged when it happens; people with Avoidant Personality Disorder, however, operate on the assumption that they will be criticized. Because anyone can be hurt by especially severe criticism, it is important to establish that the amount of distress is well beyond the response of most people to similar criticism and that the person is so constantly on guard against the possibility of being criticized that he or she spends a lot of time thinking about it.

(5) is inhibited in new interpersonal situations because of feelings of inadequacy

Interviewer's Questions: You've said that you're *[Are you]* usually quiet when you meet new people. Why is that? (Is it because you feel in some way inadequate or not good enough?)

Commentary: People with this disorder tend to be silent and "invisible," particularly in new situations, because they feel that anything they say will be "wrong" or will reveal their inadequacy.

(6) views self as socially inept, personally unappealing, or inferior to others

Interviewer's Questions: You've said that *[Do]* you believe that you're not as good, as smart, or as attractive as most other people. Tell me about that.

Commentary: The pervasive low self-esteem of people with this disorder is evident in the various ways they put themselves down. They may unrealistically believe that they are ugly or stupid and that they always do or say the wrong thing in social situations.

(7) is unusually reluctant to take personal risks or to engage in any new activities because they may prove embarrassing

Interviewer's Questions: You've said that you're *[Are you]* afraid to try new things. Is that because you are afraid of being embarrassed? Give me some examples.

Commentary: In some people with Avoidant Personality Disorder, their avoidance becomes such a generalized phenomenon that they refuse to do anything outside of their normal routine. They may see any new project or activity only as an opportunity to reveal how inept, ugly, or otherwise unworthy they are. They may therefore avoid job interviews, classes, or learning how to do anything new, from skiing to computer programming, for fear of doing it wrong.

5.2 Dependent Personality Disorder

(1) has difficulty making everyday decisions without an excessive amount of advice and reassurance from others

Interviewer's Questions: You've said that *[Do]* you need a lot of advice or reassurance from others before you can make everyday decisions—like what to wear or what to order in a restaurant. Can you give me some examples of the kinds of decisions you would ask for advice or reassurance about? (Does this happen most of the time?)

Commentary: People with Dependent Personality Disorder need others to make decisions for them. This item refers to an inability to make everyday decisions (for example, deciding which clothes to wear in the morning, making a selection from a menu) rather than major decisions (whether to get married, where to live), which are covered by the next item. This personality trait must be differentiated from indecisiveness (a feature of Major Depressive Episode), in which the primary pathology is an inability to make decisions rather than the need to rely on others for help in making them.

(2) needs others to assume responsibility for most major areas of his or her life

Interviewer's Questions: You've said that you *[Do you]* depend on other people to handle important areas in your life such as finances, child care, or living arrangements. Give me some examples. (Is this more than just getting advice from people?) (Has this happened with MOST important areas of your life?)

Commentary: People with Dependent Personality Disorder typically allow and even encourage others to make important life decisions for them. Such decisions include selection of friends, schools, careers, employment, spouse, place to live, and the like. Seeking advice about such decisions is normal and by itself does not constitute sufficient evidence to warrant a rating of "3." The person must clearly *defer* the decisions to other people. Use careful clinical judgment when considering this question for adolescents and young adults, making allowances for age-appropriate dependence on parents or parental surrogates. Also, be sure to take subcultural norms (e.g., arranged marriages) into account in rating this item.

(3) has difficulty expressing disagreement with others because of fear of loss of support or approval (**Note:** Do not include realistic fears of retribution.)

Interviewer's Questions: You've said that *[Do]* you find it hard to disagree with people even when you think they are wrong. Give me some examples of when you've found it hard to disagree. What are you afraid will happen if you disagree?

Commentary: Passivity and being subjugated often are characteristic features of Dependent Personality Disorder; they may manifest themselves in attempts to be excessively agreeable, with the goal of being liked. To warrant a rating of "3," this behavior should not be limited to interactions with people of a higher rank or status (e.g., bosses or professors).

(4) has difficulty initiating projects or doing things on his or her own (because of a lack of self-confidence in judgment or abilities rather than a lack of motivation or energy)

Interviewer's Questions: You've said *[Do]* you find it hard to start or work on tasks when there is no one to help you. Give me some examples. Why is that? (Is this because you are not sure you can do it right?)

Commentary: Because of their excessive reliance on the advice and support of others, people with Dependent Personality Disorder avoid working on their own or taking the initiative in starting projects or tasks. Evidence supporting a "yes" answer should be restricted to tasks that ordinarily could be accomplished without the help of other people. Be sure to establish that this overreliance on others is not limited to periods of depression.

(5) goes to excessive lengths to obtain nurturance and support from others, to the point of volunteering to do things that are unpleasant

Interviewer's Questions: You've said that you have *[Have you]* often volunteered to do things that are unpleasant. Give me some examples of these kinds of things. Why is that?

Commentary: People with Dependent Personality Disorder typically subjugate their own needs to the needs of others so that others will like them. This behavior can be so extreme that they will even volunteer to do unpleasant or demeaning things—for example, volunteering to clean toilets or getting up at dawn to wait in line for concert tickets.

(6) feels uncomfortable or helpless when alone because of exaggerated fears of being unable to care for himself or herself

Interviewer's Questions: You've said that *[Do]* you usually feel uncomfortable when you are by yourself. Why is that? (Is it because you need someone to take care of you?)

Commentary: In severe cases of Dependent Personality Disorder, the dependence on others becomes so extreme that the person experiences distress when alone even for a few hours and therefore will go to great lengths to avoid being alone. When forced to be alone, he or she may make repeated urgent phone calls to "caretakers." Note that people with Borderline Personality Disorder also can become distressed when alone. The difference is that, in Dependent Personality Disorder, the person's primary concern is that he or she does not have the requisite skills to take care of him or herself, whereas in Borderline Personality Disorder, the concern is that the person will "fall apart" if he or she is alone.

(7) urgently seeks another relationship as a source of care and support when a close relationship ends

Interviewer's Questions: You've said that when a close relationship ends you *[When a close relationship ends, do you]* feel you immediately have to find someone else to take care of you. Tell me about that. (Have you reacted this way almost always when close relationships have ended?)

Commentary: Although most people feel upset when a close relationship ends, people with Dependent Personality Disorder are overwhelmed by the loss and often urgently seek an immediate replacement for the lost person. They may become quickly and indiscriminately attached to another person because they feel unable to care for themselves. (An inability to function due to a Major Depressive Disorder initiated by a breakup or impairment in functioning during a period of bereavement does not constitute evidence supporting a rating of "3" for this item.)

(8) is unrealistically preoccupied with fears of being left to take care of himself or herself

Interviewer's Questions: You've said that *[Do]* you worry a lot about being left alone to take care of yourself. Are there often times when you keep worrying about this? Do you have periods when you worry about this all the time?

Commentary: People with Dependent Personality Disorder often become preoccupied with the fear of being abandoned because of their feeling that they cannot cope by themselves, even when there is no real threat of abandonment. This item should not be rated "3" if the evidence is limited to particular circumstances, such as the impending death of a loved one, or if the fear of abandonment is a realistic concern (e.g., an elderly person with no surviving friends or family or a person with a disabling physical illness).

5.3 Obsessive-Compulsive Personality Disorder

(1) is preoccupied with details, rules, lists, order, organization, or schedules to the extent that the major point of the activity is lost

Interviewer's Questions: You've said that you are *[Are you]* the kind of person who focuses on details, order, and organization or likes to make lists and schedules. Give me some examples. Do you sometimes get so caught up with [EXAMPLES] that you lose sight of what you are trying to accomplish? (. . . like you can't see the forest for the trees?) (Does this happen often?)

Commentary: People with Obsessive-Compulsive Personality Disorder are overly concerned with the details, process, or method of accomplishing a task. When this is extreme, so much time is spent focusing on these details that they become ends in themselves and the task is prolonged, completed only partially, or not completed at all. Although this pattern usually is most relevant in occupational situations (e.g., with projects at work) or housework, it may occur in other settings; an individual may become so preoccupied with planning the minute details of a trip that he or she is unable to enjoy the trip itself.

(2) shows perfectionism that interferes with task completion (e.g., is unable to complete a project because his or her own overly strict standards are not met)

Interviewer's Questions: You've said that *[Do]* you have trouble finishing jobs because you spend so much time trying to get things exactly right. Give me some examples. (How often does this happen?)

Commentary: Perfectionism is a trait that often results in occupational productivity and success. This item should be rated "3" only if there is evidence that the perfectionism is so pronounced that it interferes with task completion: either tasks are never completed because of the insistence on getting things exactly right or they are significantly delayed. This item differs from the previous item in that the impairment in functioning is related to perfectionism rather than (or in addition to) getting lost in the details.

(3) is excessively devoted to work and productivity to the exclusion of leisure activities and friendships (not accounted for by obvious economic necessity)

Interviewer's Questions: You've said that you or other people feel that you *[Do you or other people feel that you]* are so devoted to work (or school) that you have no time left for anyone else or for just having fun. Tell me about it.

Commentary: This item should be rated "3" if the person is so dedicated to his or her work that there is virtually no time left for the pursuit of leisure activities (e.g., no hobbies and never attends sports, concerts, movies, etc.) or interpersonal relationships (e.g., never spends time with spouse, children, or friends). The person may provide rationalizations for this behavior (e.g., "I love my work," "It's important so I can get ahead," "I can't get all my work done during the day"), but the only explanations that should result in a rating of "1" would be those involving obvious economic necessity (for example, working a second job to provide basic support for family) or special short-term circumstances (such as a brief period of long work hours prior to a deadline, or a medical internship).

(4) is overconscientious, scrupulous, and inflexible about matters of morality, ethics, or values (not accounted for by cultural or religious identification)

Interviewer's Questions: You've said that *[Do]* you have very high standards about what is right and what is wrong. Give me some examples of your high standards. (Do you follow rules to the letter of the law, no matter what?) IF GIVES RELIGIOUS EXAMPLE: Do even people who share your religious views say you're too strict about right and wrong?

Commentary: This question concerns the tendency of people with Obsessive-Compulsive Personality Disorder to extend their inflexible nature and concern with high standards to the arena of morality and ethics. Many people believe they have higher moral standards than others. This item should be coded "3" only if there is evidence that the person is overly conscientious, rigid, scrupulous, or self-righteous. Such individuals have an excessive concern about doing what is right and may be very worried about having done something wrong. It is important to consider the cultural and religious background of the person because this behavior often appears in a religious context—the item should be coded "3" only if he or she is considerably more inflexible or conscientious than others sharing the same religious or cultural background. An example would be someone who chastises friends for engaging in harmless gossip.

(5) is unable to discard worn-out or worthless objects even when they have no sentimental value

> *Interviewer's Questions:* You've said that *[Do]* you have trouble throwing things out because they might come in handy some day. Give me some examples of things that you're unable to throw out. (How cluttered does your place get because you don't throw things out?)

Commentary: Because people so commonly save things in case they are needed in the future, this item should be rated "3" only if the behavior is clearly pathological. People with this trait save things that they are extremely unlikely to use again (i.e., numerous plastic containers or corks, many years worth of newspapers and magazines, etc.) Difficulty throwing away only things that have some special personal importance (like classroom notes from junior high school) is not evidence that the trait is present. In addition, to justify a rating of "3" the end result of this behavior should cause a problem for the person (i.e., the trait must result in a cluttered environment that makes it difficult for the person to find things he or she needs, or the behavior is distressing to others who share the environment).

(6) is reluctant to delegate tasks or to work with others unless they submit to exactly his or her way of doing things

> *Interviewer's Questions:* You've said that it is *[Is it]* hard for you to let other people help you unless they agree to do things exactly the way you want. Tell me about that. (Does this happen often?) (Do you often end up doing things yourself to make sure they are done right?)

Commentary: People with Obsessive-Compulsive Personality Disorder characteristically insist that things always be done their way. Because of extensive rationalization, establishing that the person's insistence is truly "unreasonable" may be difficult; the person may provide plausible explanations that lend credence to the contention that his or her way is indeed the best. In these cases, evidence should be culled from the person's stubbornness in activities in which the "best way" is debatable, such as household cleaning tasks. Often there will have been complaints from others about the person's bossiness; frequently a person with this characteristic ends up doing things himself or herself to be sure they are done the "right" way.

(7) adopts a miserly spending style toward both self and others; money is viewed as something to be hoarded for future catastrophes

> *Interviewer's Questions:* You've said that it is *[Is it]* hard for you to spend money on yourself and other people even when you have enough. Why? (Is this because you're worried about not having enough in the future when you really need it?) Tell me about some things you haven't spent money on because you have to save for the future.

Commentary: The personality trait of generosity manifests itself on a continuum, ranging from self-sacrificing to stingy. This item should be rated "3" only if the person is clearly much less generous than most others would be in comparable circumstances.

(8) shows rigidity and stubbornness

> *Interviewer's Questions:* You've said that you are *[Are you]* often so sure you are right that it doesn't matter what other people say. Tell me

about it. You've said that other people have told you *[Have other people told you]* that you are stubborn or rigid. Tell me about that.

Commentary: Totally wrapped up in their own perspective, people with this disorder have difficulty acknowledging the viewpoints of others or going along with anyone else's ideas. Even when they recognize that it may be in their interest to compromise, they may stubbornly refuse to do so, arguing that it is "the principle of the thing."

5.4 Passive-Aggressive Personality Disorder

(1) passively resists fulfilling routine social and occupational tasks

Interviewer's Questions: You've said that when someone asks you to do something that you don't want to do, you *[When someone asks you to do something that you don't want to do, do you]* say "yes" but then work slowly or do a bad job. Give me some examples of this. You've said that if you don't want to do something you *[If you don't want to do something, do you]* often just "forget" to do it. Give me some examples of this.

Commentary: The behavior described here is the essence of the passive-aggressive nature; aggressive impulses take the form of passive resistance to demands for adequate performance. Passive resistance can take many forms and occurs in both social and occupational settings: for example, saying "yes" when the person means "no"; "forgetting" to do tasks or assignments that the person does not want to do; doing assignments halfheartedly and sloppily and being intentionally inefficient; chronically arriving hours late to family functions; or not showing up at social engagements after responding that he or she will attend. In some cases, these people may hide behind perfectionism, attributing their nonperformance of a task to concerns about doing it correctly.

(2) complains of being misunderstood and unappreciated by others

Interviewer's Questions: You've said that *[Do]* you often feel that other people don't understand you or don't appreciate how much you do. Tell me more about that. (Do you complain to other people about this?)

Commentary: People with this trait overvalue their own role in any endeavor and do not understand why other people do not give them more credit. To justify a rating of "3," the person must have actively complained to others about this.

(3) is sullen and argumentative

Interviewer's Questions: You've said that you're *[Are you]* often grumpy and likely to get into arguments. Tell me when this happens.

Commentary: People with this trait feel put upon, oppressed, and long-suffering and often are resentfully silent, irritable, impatient, skeptical, or contrary. Any ordinary request is perceived as an undue burden on their time and energy and is likely to elicit an argument. Other people may simply stop asking anything of this person because getting them to participate or contribute is not worth the argument.

(4) unreasonably criticizes and scorns authority

Interviewer's Questions: You've said that you've *[Have you]* found that most of your bosses, teachers, supervisors, doctors, and others who are supposed to know what they are doing really don't. Tell me about that.

Commentary: People with this trait rarely have respect for anyone in authority, viewing them as demanding, incompetent, negligent, or uncaring. Because of their tendency to externalize blame, they will criticize authority figures with minimal provocation.

(5) expresses envy and resentment toward those apparently more fortunate

Interviewer's Questions: You've said that *[Do]* you often think that it's not fair that other people have more than you do. Tell me more about that.

Commentary: This characteristic often is expressed in a litany of complaints that those who are better off in some way (e.g., wealthier or more prominent) don't deserve it.

(6) voices exaggerated and persistent complaints of personal misfortune

Interviewer's Questions: You've said that *[Do]* you often complain that more than your share of bad things have happened to you. Looking back on your life, do you feel that bad things are always happening to you?

Commentary: Because of the difficulty in determining whether a particular complaint is in fact exaggerated, a rating of "3" should be given only if the person complains of lifelong and persistent personal misfortune.

(7) alternates between hostile defiance and contrition

Interviewer's Questions: You've said that *[Do]* you often angrily refuse to do what others want and then later feel bad and apologize. Tell me more about this.

Commentary: After expressing hostile defiance, the person then protects himself or herself from retaliation by obsequious apologies and promises to perform better in the future.

5.5 Depressive Personality Disorder

Commentary: Criterion B of the research criteria for Depressive Personality Disorder indicates that the diagnosis should be made ONLY if the depressive cognition and behavior "does not occur exclusively during Major Depressive Episodes and is not better accounted for by Dysthymic Disorder." This criterion was included to prevent overuse of this research diagnosis and encourage instead the use of an established diagnosis, i.e., Dysthymic Disorder. Because the relationship between Dysthymic Disorder and Depressive Personality Disorder is a research question, researchers may wish to suspend the criterion and diagnose both Depressive Personality Disorder and Dysthymic Disorder if the criteria for each are met. Alternatively, Depressive Personality Disorder may be diagnosed comorbidly with Dysthymic Disorder if the criteria are met for Depressive Personality Disorder at times other than when the full criteria are met for Dysthymic Disorder (e.g., periods in which the vegetative symptoms like overeating and insomnia are not present).

(1) usual mood is dominated by dejection, gloominess, cheerlessness, joylessness, unhappiness

Interviewer's Questions: You've said that *[Do]* you usually feel unhappy or like life is no fun. Tell me about that.

Commentary: This item is equivalent to criterion A for Major Depressive Episode (i.e., "depressed mood" or "markedly diminished interest or pleasure in all, or almost all, activities"), expressed as a lifelong trait. People with this trait are overly serious, humorless, and unable to enjoy life or have a good time.

(2) self-concept centers around beliefs of inadequacy, worthlessness, and low self-esteem

Interviewer's Questions: You've said that *[Do]* you believe that you are basically an inadequate person and often don't feel good about yourself. Tell me about that.

Commentary: Most people have periods of self-doubt. To justify a rating of "3," the person must identify himself or herself as inadequate, worthless, or a failure.

(3) is critical, blaming, and derogatory toward self

Interviewer's Questions: You've said that you *[Do you]* often put yourself down. Tell me about that. (Do you often blame yourself for things that haven't worked out?)

Commentary: This item is a more severe version of the previous item. In addition to feelings of worthlessness, the person actively berates himself or herself for failures, inadequacies, or not living up to standards.

(4) is brooding and given to worry

Interviewer's Questions: You've said that *[Do]* you keep thinking about bad things that have happened in the past or worry about bad things that might happen in the future. Tell me about that.

Commentary: People with this trait dwell on their negative and pessimistic thoughts and worry about anticipated negative consequences. The source of these feelings may be the person's doubts about his or her ability to make the right decisions.

(5) is negativistic, critical, and judgmental toward others

Interviewer's Questions: You've said that *[Do]* you often judge others harshly and easily find fault with them. Give me some examples of the kinds of things you are critical of. You've said that you *[Do you]* think that most people are basically no good. Tell me about that.

Commentary: People with this disorder often turn their hypercriticalness to the outside world and judge other people as harshly as they judge themselves.

(6) is pessimistic

Interviewer's Questions: You've said that you *[Do you]* almost always expect things to turn out badly. Tell me about that.

Commentary: This item reflects a common fundamental distortion in one's perception of oneself and the world. People with this trait always perceive the glass as "half-empty" rather than "half-full." They often rationalize their pessimistic perspective as being "realistic."

(7) is prone to feeling guilty or remorseful

Interviewer's Questions: You've said that you *[Do you]* often feel guilty about things you have or haven't done. What kinds of things?

Commentary: People with this trait take credit for everything that has ever gone wrong and then end up feeling guilty and remorseful.

5.6 Paranoid Personality Disorder

(1) suspects, without sufficient basis, that others are exploiting, harming, or deceiving him or her

Interviewer's Questions: You've said that *[Do]* you often have to keep an eye out to stop people from using you or hurting you. Tell me about that.

Commentary: This item expresses the core feature of the disorder—namely, a fundamental expectation that others will exploit, take advantage of, or hurt the person. When trying to make an assessment of this item, the focus should be on establishing a general paranoid orientation, in addition to looking for specific examples of paranoid ideation.

(2) is preoccupied with unjustified doubts about the loyalty or trustworthiness of friends or associates

Interviewer's Questions: You've said that you *[Do you]* spend a lot of time wondering if you can trust your friends or the people you work with. Describe situations where you've gotten that feeling. (Do you feel this way often?)

Commentary: Because determining whether a lack of trust is unjustified in a particular case often is very difficult, the item should be rated "3" only if the person is preoccupied with these kinds of doubts in almost all relationships. This item differs from the previous one in that item 1 reflects a general paranoid perspective about the environment, whereas this item reflects the person's expectations of betrayal even by family, friends, or co-workers.

(3) is reluctant to confide in others because of unwarranted fear that the information will be used maliciously against him or her

> *Interviewer's Questions:* You've said that *[Do]* you find that it is best not to let other people know much about you because they will use it against you. When has this happened? Tell me about it.

Commentary: It is important to determine that the reason for the individual's reluctance to confide in others is a fear of some harm resulting from having confided the information, rather than merely a fear of rejection (which is characteristic of Avoidant Personality Disorder). In addition, this item should not be coded "3" if the reluctance to confide in a particular person seems justified based on previous experience with that person.

(4) reads hidden demeaning or threatening meanings into benign remarks or events

> *Interviewer's Questions:* You've said that *[Do]* you often detect hidden threats or insults in things people say or do. Give me some examples.

Commentary: This characteristic consists of idiosyncratic personalized interpretations of innocuous behavior as having a malevolent intent. This trait is the "paranoid" version of item 1 in Schizotypal Personality Disorder, in which an event or object in the person's environment has a particular or unusual significance. To be coded "3" for Paranoid Personality Disorder, the ideas of reference must have a threatening or demeaning content.

(5) persistently bears grudges (i.e., is unforgiving of insults, injuries, or slights)

> *Interviewer's Questions:* You've said that you're *[Are you]* the kind of person who holds grudges or takes a long time to forgive people who have insulted or slighted you. Tell me about that. You've said that there are *[Are there]* many people you can't forgive because they did or said something to you a long time ago. Tell me about that.

Commentary: To qualify as a "grudge," the person's reaction must be clearly out of proportion to the severity or intensity of the insult or injury. For example, a lifelong grudge against a person for murdering a friend would not be out of proportion, but refusal to speak to a close friend for several years after a minor argument would be.

(6) perceives attacks on his or her character or reputation that are not apparent to others and is quick to react angrily or to counterattack

> *Interviewer's Questions:* You've said that *[Do]* you often get angry or lash out when someone criticizes or insults you in some way. Give me some examples. (Do others believe that you often take offense too easily?)

Commentary: There are two parts to this item. First, the person must be hypersensitive to minor insults, indignities, or omissions. Second (and distinguishing this from the "is preoccupied by criticism" item under Avoidant Personality Disorder), the person is quick to react with anger or counterattack.

(7) has recurrent suspicions, without justification, regarding fidelity of spouse or sexual partner

> *Interviewer's Questions:* You've said that you have *[Have you]* often suspected that your spouse or partner has been unfaithful. Tell me about that. (What clues did you have? What did you do about it? Were you right?)

Commentary: The usual difficulty in assessing this item is determining whether or not the jealousy is "pathological"—that is, persistent and unjustified.

This often requires careful questioning or establishing frequent instances of jealousy occurring in several different relationships. Excessive and inappropriate behavior often is associated with the jealousy, such as neglecting other responsibilities to monitor a spouse's (or lover's) activities.

5.7 Schizotypal Personality Disorder

(1) ideas of reference (excluding delusions of reference)

> *Interviewer's Questions:* You've said that when you are out in public and see people talking *[When you are out in public and see people talking, do]* you often feel that they are talking about you. Tell me more about this. You've said that you *[Do you]* often get the feeling that things that have no special meaning to most people are really meant to give you a message. Tell me more about this. You've said that when you are around people, you *[When you are around people, do you]* often get the feeling that you are being watched or stared at. Tell me more about this.

Commentary: Ideas of reference (also known as referential thinking) are typical of the ideation that is characteristic of this personality disorder. A person with an idea of reference has the belief that an event, object, or other person in the immediate environment has a particular or unusual significance to him or her. A common example is a person who often has the feeling that when he sees a group of strangers talking to each other, they are talking about him. Much less common is the person who believes objects in the environment contain a special message. For example, a woman named Gloria interprets a sign on a nut store that says "Gloria's Nuts" as a message that she is crazy. An idea of reference should be distinguished from a delusion of reference, in which the referential idea is held with delusional intensity (i.e., the person firmly believes that the delusion of reference is true and will not seriously entertain alternate explanations). In cases in which the referential thinking reaches delusional proportions, a diagnosis of a psychotic disorder (on Axis I) should be seriously considered.

(2) odd beliefs or magical thinking that influences behavior and is inconsistent with subcultural norms (e.g., superstitiousness, belief in clairvoyance, telepathy, or "sixth sense"; in children and adolescents, bizarre fantasies or preoccupations)

> *Interviewer's Questions:* You've said that you have *[Have you ever]* felt that you could make things happen just by making a wish or thinking about them. Tell me about that. (How did it affect you?) You've said that you have *[Have you]* had personal experiences with the supernatural. Tell me about that. (How did it affect you?) You've said that you *[Do you]* believe that you have a "sixth sense" that allows you to know and predict things that others can't. Tell me about that. (How does it affect you?)

Commentary: Some superstitions and other beliefs that are not consistent with the laws of nature and physics are common in most societies and cultures. To qualify for this item, the person must do more than just acknowledge having such beliefs by reporting some influence of these beliefs on his or her behavior. For example, a person who just reports believing in the existence of ESP should not be rated "3" on this item; instead, the person must report a personal experience with ESP that influenced his or her behavior. In addition, this criterion should be considered only for beliefs that deviate considerably from the norms of the person's subculture. Magical thinking is a particular kind of "odd belief" in which the person believes that his or her words, thoughts, or actions will cause something to occur or prevent something from occurring in a way that violates the physical laws of cause and effect. An example is a person believing that his intense wish to win the lottery was responsible for his winning. Note that, by definition, magical thinking is nondelusional in that the person believes the idea with less than delusional intensity—that is, the person can entertain the possibility of alternate explanations. (The requirement that the belief be of less than delusional intensity applies to this entire criterion.)

(3) unusual perceptual experiences, including bodily illusions

> *Interviewer's Questions:* You've said that it often seems *[Does it often seem]* that objects or shadows are really people or animals or that noises are actually people's voices. Give me some examples. (Were you drinking or taking drugs at the time?) You've said that you have *[Have you]* had the sense that some person or force is around you, even though you cannot see anyone. Tell me more about that. (Were you drinking or taking drugs at the time?) You've said that you *[Do you]* often see auras or energy fields around people. Tell me more about that. (Were you drinking or taking drugs at the time?)

Commentary: This item should be rated "3" if there are unusual perceptual experiences other than nontransient hallucinations, which would suggest the presence of a psychotic disorder. In addition, unusual perceptual experiences that are due to drugs (e.g., hallucinogens), physical disorders (e.g., metabolic encephalopathy), or natural phenomena (e.g., hypnagogic or hypnopompic hallucinations that occur upon falling asleep or awakening from sleep) should not be considered evidence for this criterion.

(4) odd thinking and speech (e.g., vague, circumstantial, metaphorical, over-elaborate, or stereotyped)

Commentary: This behavior is observed during the interview. Other examples of odd speech include idiosyncratic word usage; neologisms; speech with no content; and stilted, overly concrete, or overly tangential speech. Note that speech that is so disordered that it is classifiable as "loosening of associations" or "incoherence" suggests a diagnosis of Schizophrenia.

(5) suspiciousness or paranoid ideation

Commentary: This item should be coded "3" if any of Paranoid Personality Disorder criteria 1, 2, 3, 4, or 7 have been coded "3." The relevant items in Paranoid Personality Disorder are: (1) suspects, without sufficient basis, that others are exploiting, harming, or deceiving him or her; (2) is preoccupied with unjustified doubts about the loyalty or trustworthiness of friends or associates; (3) is reluctant to confide in others because of unwarranted fear that the information will be used maliciously against him or her; (4) reads hidden demeaning or threatening meanings into benign remarks or events; and (7) has recurrent suspicions, without justification, regarding fidelity of spouse or sexual partner.

(6) inappropriate or constricted affect

Commentary: This behavior is observed during the interview. Inappropriate affect is defined as an incongruity between the content of what the person is saying and his or her vocal inflections and facial expression. It often is expressed as inappropriate cheerfulness (e.g., smiling brightly when telling about something terrible that happened). Do not include inappropriate laughter that is due to anxiety. Evidence for constricted affect includes unchanging facial expression, monotonous or unvarying vocal inflection, absence of expressive gestures, keeping a rigid posture, and poor eye contact. Any evidence of constricted affect must be present over a prolonged period of time and should clearly not be caused by depressed mood or medication effects (e.g., neuroleptics).

(7) behavior or appearance that is odd, eccentric, or peculiar

Commentary: This behavior or appearance is observed during the interview. Examples of odd behavior should be present over a prolonged period of time and not caused by some other mental disorder (e.g., Manic Episode or Schizophrenia). Examples would include talking to oneself in the street, wearing items of clothing that obviously do not fit together, or wearing many layers of clothing on a warm day. This item is not meant however, to apply to individuals who dress in an unusual way simply to be stylish.

(8) lack of close friends or confidants other than first-degree relatives

> *Interviewer's Questions:* You've said that there are *[Are there]* very few people that you're really close to outside of your immediate family. How many close friends do you have?

Commentary: People with Schizoid and Schizotypal Personality Disorders typically have very few friends or confidants; they tend to avoid close relationships with other people, albeit for different reasons. People with Schizoid Personality Disorder avoid close friendships because they have little interest in relationships with other people. Those with Schizotypal Personality Disorder feel uncomfortable in relationships because of excessive social anxiety and social awkwardness, and therefore avoid such relationships.

(9) excessive social anxiety that does not diminish with familiarity and tends to be associated with paranoid fears rather than negative judgments about self

> *Interviewer's Questions:* You've said that *[Do]* you often feel nervous when you are with other people. What are you nervous about? (Are you still anxious even after you've known them for awhile?)

Commentary: A rating of "3" for this item requires that the person be much more uncomfortable than most people are in social situations, even with familiar people. The social anxiety in Schizotypal Personality Disorder is rooted in a fundamental inability to relate to other people. For this reason, familiarity does not provide reassurance and comfort. In contrast, in Avoidant Personality Disorder, familiarity reduces anxiety because it alleviates the fear of humiliation and rejection that is most relevant in the initial stages of a relationship.

5.8 Schizoid Personality Disorder

(1) neither desires nor enjoys close relationships, including being part of a family

> *Interviewer's Questions:* You've said that it is *[Is it]* NOT important to you whether you have any close relationships. Tell me more about that. (What about your family?)

Commentary: This lack of strong desire for relationships is the hallmark of Schizoid Personality Disorder and is what differentiates it from Avoidant Personality Disorder, in which the person's lack of close relationships relates to excessive social anxiety.

(2) almost always chooses solitary activities

> *Interviewer's Questions:* You've said that you would *[Would you]* almost always rather do things alone than with other people. (Is that true both at work and during your free time?)

Commentary: Because a person with this disorder has little desire for relationships, it follows that he or she would almost always choose solitary activities rather than activities that involve other people. This preference should be pervasive and extend to both work and leisure activities.

(3) has little, if any, interest in having sexual experiences with another person

> *Interviewer's Questions:* You've said that you could *[Could you]* be content without ever being sexually involved with anyone. Tell me more about that. (Have you always had little interest in having sex?)

Commentary: The lack of desire to have sexual experiences with another person must have been present since adolescence and should not be motivated simply by a fear of rejection.

(4) takes pleasure in few, if any, activities

> *Interviewer's Questions:* You've said that there are *[Are there]* really very few things that give you pleasure. Tell me about that. (What about physical things like eating a good meal or having sex?)

Commentary: Although some people with this disorder may derive pleasure from solitary intellectual activities (e.g., stamp collecting or doing mathematical problems), they generally lack the ability to take pleasure in interpersonal activities or sensory experiences (e.g., eating or sex).

(5) lacks close friends or confidants other than first-degree relatives

> [ALREADY CODED ON ITEM 8 FOR SCHIZOTYPAL PERSONALITY DISORDER]

(6) appears indifferent to the praise or criticism of others

> *Interviewer's Questions:* You've said that it doesn't *[Does it NOT]* matter to you what people think of you. How do you feel when people praise you or criticize you?

Commentary: People with this trait have little interest in relationships with other people and therefore do not care what other people think about them.

(7) shows emotional coldness, detachment, or flattened affectivity

> *Interviewer's Questions:* You've said that *[Do]* you find that nothing makes you very happy or very sad. Tell me more about that.

Commentary: Behavior that can be directly observed should be the primary basis for rating this item. People with this trait rarely show any expression of emotion, will speak in a monotone without varying their vocal inflection, and will show little or no facial expression. The interviewer must ascertain that the person characteristically appears this way (either by asking the person directly or by checking with other informants) and that this constricted affect is not due to depressed mood or the effects of medication (e.g., neuroleptics).

5.9 Histrionic Personality Disorder

(1) is uncomfortable in situations in which he or she is not the center of attention

> *Interviewer's Questions:* You've said that *[Do]* you like to be the center of attention. How do you feel when you're not?

Commentary: The desire to be noticed and have other people pay attention is normal. In Histrionic Personality Disorder, this desire for attention is so extreme that it becomes insatiable. Because the person feels uncomfortable when not the center of attention, he or she will go to great lengths to ensure being and remaining at the center, such as monopolizing conversations in a group of people or flamboyantly dramatizing story after story.

(2) interaction with others is often characterized by inappropriate sexually seductive or provocative behavior

> *Interviewer's Questions:* You've said that *[Do]* you flirt a lot. Has anyone complained about this? You've said that you *[Do you]* often find yourself "coming on" to people. Tell me about it.

Commentary: This item should be rated "3" if there are striking examples of seductive behavior that is compulsive or indiscriminate—that is, at times or in situations not related to dating, courtship, and romance. An example is someone who is flirtatious with waiters or waitresses, grocery clerks, delivery people, or the like.

(3) displays rapidly shifting and shallow expression of emotions

Commentary: This behavior is observed during the interview. This item refers to rapid shifts in expressed mood that reflect the fundamental superficiality of the affect. For example, the person might get very excited about something or someone and then quickly lose interest, or throw a temper tantrum that immediately dissipates when the person's attention shifts to something else. The person's emotions are turned on and off so quickly that others may accuse the person of faking the feelings. This is distinguished from item 6 in Borderline Personality Disorder ("affective instability") in that the shifting emotions in Borderline Personality Disorder are deeper and more sustained (i.e., lasting for hours or days).

(4) consistently uses physical appearance to draw attention to self

> *Interviewer's Questions:* You've said that you *[Do you]* try to draw attention to yourself by the way you dress or look. How do you do that? Do you do that all the time?

Commentary: This item refers to the use of physical appearance and dress as a way of defining oneself and standing out from the crowd. Do not include people whose unusual physical appearance is exclusively oppositional in nature (e.g., wearing multiple nose rings as a way of rejecting parental values).

(5) has a style of speech that is excessively impressionistic and lacking in detail

Commentary: This behavior is observed during the interview. Along with overly dramatic presentation, a person with Histrionic Personality Disorder may use a style of speech that is excessively impressionistic and is characterized by the frequent use of broad, sweeping, global statements, lacking in detail. For example, the person may describe someone as "horrible" or "wonderful" without being able to provide any supporting facts or details.

(6) shows self-dramatization, theatricality, and exaggerated expression of emotion

> *Interviewer's Questions:* You've said that you *[Do you]* often make a point of being dramatic and colorful. Tell me about that. (Do you like to show your emotions—for example, hugging people even if you don't know them very well or crying very easily?)

Commentary: People with this disorder tend to be very dramatic in telling stories about themselves or in expressing their emotions. They may embarrass friends and acquaintances by an excessive public display of emotions (e.g., embracing casual acquaintances with excessive ardor, sobbing uncontrollably on minor sentimental occasions, or having temper tantrums). This question often can be answered by observing the person's behavior during your assessment interview. Be careful not to include behavior that occurs only during Manic Episodes or Hypomanic Episodes.

(7) is suggestible (i.e., easily influenced by others or circumstances)

> *Interviewer's Questions:* You've said that you *[Do you]* often change your mind about things depending on the people you're with or what you have just read or seen on TV. Tell me more about that.

Commentary: People with this characteristic tend to follow the latest fad, adopt new convictions easily, and quickly develop new "heroes." Their opinions and values are overly influenced by their peers, co-workers, family, and media. They appear to have no stable core of their own beliefs and values.

(8) considers relationships to be more intimate than they actually are

Interviewer's Questions: You've said that you *[Do you]* have lots of friends that you are very close to. How many? Who are they?

Commentary: This characteristic may be evident in the individual's description of people he or she has just met, or had a single conversation with, as close friends.

5.10 Narcissistic Personality Disorder

(1) has a grandiose sense of self-importance (e.g., exaggerates achievements and talents, expects to be recognized as superior without commensurate achievements)

Interviewer's Questions: You've said that *[Do]* people often fail to appreciate your very special talents or accomplishments. Give me an example. You've said that people have *[Have people]* told you that you have too high an opinion of yourself. Give me some examples of this.

Commentary: Look for discrepancies between the person's expectation of recognition and his or her willingness to work or pass through ordinary hurdles (e.g., to get the required degree or go up through the ranks).

(2) is preoccupied with fantasies of unlimited success, power, brilliance, beauty, or ideal love

Interviewer's Questions: You've said that *[Do]* you think a lot about the power, fame, or recognition that will be yours someday. Tell me more about this. (How much time do you spend thinking about these things?) You've said that *[Do]* you think a lot about the perfect romance that will be yours someday. Tell me more about this. (How much time do you spend thinking about this?)

Commentary: In some people, this characteristic may be manifested by frequent daydreaming or other nonproductive activity that occurs in lieu of taking concrete steps toward reaching his or her aspirations for success, power, or love: for example, a person who spends hours sitting around in a coffee shop talking about one day being a great novelist instead of spending the time writing. In others, there may be preoccupation with activities that are ultimately fruitless because of the unachievable nature of the fantasies (e.g., a person who goes to singles bars every night looking for the perfect romance).

(3) believes that he or she is "special" and unique and can only be understood by, or should associate with, other special or high-status people (or institutions)

Interviewer's Questions: You've said that when you have a problem, *[When you have a problem, do]* you almost always insist on seeing the top person. Give me some examples. (Why do you have to see the top person?) You've said that *[Do]* you feel it is important to spend time with people who are special or influential. Why is that?

Commentary: People with Narcissistic Personality Disorder consider themselves to be special, unique, and superior to others and often will limit their contacts to others whom they consider comparably special and talented. For example, a person with Narcissistic Personality Disorder may go to a party only after being assured that other "special" people will attend as well. As a consequence of their grandiose sense of self-importance and their sense that they deserve only the best, people with Narcissistic Personality Disorder often insist on seeing only the very top person (doctor, lawyer, hairdresser, teacher) or those from the most prestigious institutions.

(4) requires excessive admiration

Interviewer's Questions: You've said that it is *[Is it]* very important to you that people pay attention to you or admire you in some way. Tell me more about this.

Commentary: The self-esteem of individuals with Narcissistic Personality Disorder invariably is very fragile and must be bolstered constantly by the attention and admiration of others. Persons with this trait may report being preoccupied with concerns about how well they are doing and how others perceive them or may report feelings of dysphoria when they are not the object of attention or admiration.

(5) has a sense of entitlement (i.e., unreasonable expectations of especially favorable treatment or automatic compliance with his or her expectations)

> *Interviewer's Questions:* You've said that *[Do]* you think that it's not necessary to follow certain rules or social conventions when they get in your way. Give me some examples. Why do you feel that way? You've said that *[Do]* you feel that you are the kind of person who deserves special treatment. Tell me more about this.

Commentary: Make sure that the expectation of special treatment is truly unreasonable, taking into account the actual status of the person. Typically, the person feels entitled to special treatment because of his or her intrinsic "specialness." For example, people with Narcisstic Personality Disorder may assume that they should not have to wait in line because their needs are so important that others should defer to them.

(6) is interpersonally exploitative (i.e., takes advantage of others to achieve his or her own ends)

> *Interviewer's Questions:* You've said that *[Do]* you often find it necessary to step on a few toes to get what you want. Tell me some instances of that. (Does that happen often?) You've said that *[Do]* you often have to put your needs above other people's. Give me some examples of when that happens. You've said that *[Do]* you often expect other people to do what you ask without question because of who you are. (Does this happen often?)

Commentary: The combination of entitlement and lack of sensitivity to the needs of others often leads to the exploitation of others. People with Narcissistic Personality Disorder feel they are so important and special that their needs deserve to be met no matter what the consequences for others. They may establish friendships or romantic relationships with others only if those relationships are likely to enhance their self-esteem or further their goals.

(7) lacks empathy: is unwilling to recognize or identify with the feelings and needs of others

> *Interviewer's Questions:* You've said that you're *[Are you]* NOT really interested in other people's problems or feelings. Tell me about that. You've said that people have *[Have people]* complained to you that you don't listen to them or care about their feelings. Tell me about that.

Commentary: People with Narcissistic Personality Disorder generally are oblivious to the concerns, needs, and welfare of others. They tend to dominate conversations, discussing their own concerns and interests in lengthy detail without regard for the feelings and needs of others. They may have the capacity to demonstrate empathy (e.g., a successful therapist with Narcissistic Personality Disorder) but only if it serves their own purposes.

(8) is often envious of others or believes that others are envious of him or her

> *Interviewer's Questions:* You've said that you are *[Are you]* often envious of others. Tell me about it. (How often do you feel that way?) You've said that *[Do]* you feel that others are often envious of you. What do they envy about you?

Commentary: People with Narcissistic Personality Disorder are constantly judging how well they measure up to others. They often devalue or denigrate others' successes, believing that they deserve the admiration or privileges themselves. In some cases, they assume that others must be envious of them.

(9) shows arrogant, haughty behaviors or attitudes

Interviewer's Questions: You've said that you *[Do you]* find that there are very few people that are worth your time and attention. Tell me about that.

Commentary: The interviewer should look for evidence of snobbish or patronizing attitudes or behaviors. These attitudes often are evident during the interview—for example, the person disdainfully comments about the interviewer's style, appearance, or the interview itself (e.g., "who thought up these stupid questions?").

5.11 Borderline Personality Disorder

(1) frantic efforts to avoid real or imagined abandonment (**Note:** Do not include suicidal or self-mutilating behavior covered in item (5).)

Interviewer's Questions: You've said that you have *[Have you]* often become frantic when you thought that someone you really cared about was going to leave you. What have you done? (Have you threatened or pleaded with him/her?)

Commentary: This item refers to frantic actions taken by the person to keep someone that they are involved with, attached to, or dependent on from leaving. Examples include pleading with someone not to leave or physically restraining the person.

(2) a pattern of unstable and intense interpersonal relationships characterized by alternating between extremes of idealization and devaluation

Interviewer's Questions: You've said that *[Do]* your relationships with people you really care about have lots of extreme ups and downs. Tell me about them. (Were there times when you thought they were everything you wanted and other times when you thought they were terrible? How many relationships were like this?)

Commentary: There are three necessary components to this criterion. First, there must be a pattern of unstable relationships, characterized by frequent conflict and threats of separation (or actual periods of separation). Second, these relationships must be intense: strong emotions (such as euphoria, infatuation, anger, resentment, or despair) must be present. Finally, the person must relate to the other person in the relationship with overidealization ("my boyfriend is the most wonderful, caring, strong person I've ever met") at times and devaluation ("he's really scum") at other times. In analytic terms, these individuals commonly use splitting as a defense mechanism.

(3) identity disturbance: markedly and persistently unstable self-image or sense of self

Interviewer's Questions: You've said that you have *[Have you]* all of a sudden changed your sense of who you are and where you are headed. Give me some examples of this. You've said that your *[Does your]* sense of who you are often changes dramatically. Tell me more about that. You've said that you are *[Are you]* different with different people or in different situations, so that you sometimes don't know who you really are. Give me some examples of this. (Do you feel this way a lot?) You've said that there have been *[Have there been]* lots of sudden changes in your goals, career plans, religious beliefs, and so on. Tell me more about that.

Commentary: Identity is a stable sense of self that provides a unity of personality over time. The type of identity disturbance that is characteristic of Borderline Personality Disorder consists of extreme shifts in the person's sense of who he or she is, which often is manifested in abrupt changes in jobs or career goals, reported sexual orientation, personal values, friends, or the person's fundamental sense of self (e.g., as evil or good). Note that this item should be rated "3" only if the identity disturbance is not appropriate for the person's developmental age (i.e., normal adolescent identity shifts should not be considered).

(4) impulsivity in at least two areas that are potentially self-damaging (e.g., spending, sex, substance abuse, reckless driving, binge eating). (**Note:** Do not include suicidal or self-mutilating behavior covered in item (5).)

> *Interviewer's Questions:* You've said that you've *[Have you]* often done things impulsively. What kinds of things? (How about buying things you really couldn't afford? having sex with people you hardly knew, or "unsafe sex"? drinking too much or taking drugs? driving recklessly? uncontrollable eating?) IF YES TO ANY OF ABOVE: Tell me about that. How often does it happen? What kinds of problems has it caused?

Commentary: The central feature of this criterion is the person's inability to exercise control over his or her impulses to engage in behavior that may be gratifying in the short run but potentially destructive in the long run. Note that the behaviors listed in the interview questions are merely examples; they are not intended to be exhaustive. In this list, "spending" refers to impulsive purchases of things the person cannot really afford, and "sex" refers to impulsively deciding to have sex with someone (or having "unsafe sex") without consideration of potentially self-damaging consequences.

(5) recurrent suicidal behavior, gestures, or threats, or self-mutilating behavior

> *Interviewer's Questions:* You've said that you have *[Have you]* tried to hurt or kill yourself or threatened to do so. You've said that you have *[Have you ever]* cut, burned, or scratched yourself on purpose. Tell me about that.

Commentary: Do not rate this item "3" for a person who simply tells others about passive suicidal ideation ("I wish I were dead"). "Self-mutilating behavior" refers to physically self-injurious behavior without any suicidal intent. Common examples include wrist-cutting or -scratching and burning oneself with a cigarette.

(6) affective instability due to a marked reactivity of mood (e.g., intense episodic dysphoria, irritability, or anxiety usually lasting a few hours and only rarely more than a few days)

> *Interviewer's Questions:* You've said that *[Do]* you have a lot of sudden mood changes. Tell me about that. (How long do your "bad" moods last? How often do these mood changes happen? How suddenly do your moods change?)

Commentary: Affective instability refers to the shifting, unstable quality of the person's mood. Although the change in mood often is abrupt, sudden onset of mood change is not a requirement. Instead, this criterion specifies frequent, large-magnitude mood changes of relatively brief duration—hours, rather than days or weeks.

(7) chronic feelings of emptiness

> *Interviewer's Questions:* You've said that *[Do]* you often feel empty inside. Tell me more about this.

Commentary: Chronic feelings of emptiness often are associated with feeling bored, hollow, alone, or without definition.

(8) inappropriate, intense anger or difficulty controlling anger (e.g., frequent displays of temper, constant anger, recurrent physical fights)

> *Interviewer's Questions:* You've said that *[Do]* you often have temper outbursts or get so angry that you lose control. Tell me about this. You've said that *[Do]* you hit people or throw things when you get angry. Tell me about this. (Does this happen often?) You've said that *[Do]* even little things get you very angry. When does this happen? (Does this happen often?)

Commentary: "Inappropriate anger" denotes that the intensity of the person's anger is out of proportion to the cause. Lack of control of anger may be evidenced by extreme physical displays such as hitting people or throwing things. The anger often is expressed in the context of real or perceived lack of caring, deprivation, or abandonment.

(9) transient, stress-related paranoid ideation or severe dissociative symptoms

> *Interviewer's Questions:* You've said that when you are under a lot of stress, you *[When you are under a lot of stress, do you]* get suspicious of other people or feel especially spaced out. Tell me about that.

Commentary: During periods of stress, some people with Borderline Personality Disorder develop transient paranoid or dissociative symptoms that are rarely severe enough to warrant an additional diagnosis (e.g., Brief Psychotic Disorder). The stressor often is real, perceived, or anticipated withdrawal of care or attention of a caregiver (e.g., lover, parent, therapist). In such situations, the real or perceived return of the caregiver's nurturance may result in a remission of the symptoms. Dissociative symptoms include periods of dissociative amnesia (e.g., having the feeling that one has lost time), depersonalization (i.e., a feeling of detachment or estrangement from one's self), or derealization (i.e., the sense that the external world is unreal or strange). These episodes typically last minutes or hours.

5.12 Antisocial Personality Disorder

Criterion B: The individual is at least age 18 years

The convention in DSM-IV is that a diagnosis of Antisocial Personality Disorder cannot be given to individuals younger than age 18. For adolescents with antisocial behavior, a diagnosis of Conduct Disorder should be considered instead.

Criterion C: Evidence of Conduct Disorder before age 15

The DSM-IV text explicating this criterion indicates that there must have been "some symptoms of Conduct Disorder before age 15" (American Psychiatric Association 1994, p. 646) without providing any indication of exactly how many are required. SCID-II operationalizes this by requiring at least two symptoms. The use of the phrase "some symptoms" implies that more than one is required, whereas a requirement of three symptoms would be at the diagnostic threshold for Conduct Disorder. That threshold clearly is higher than what was intended by the DSM-IV Childhood Disorders Work Group, which specifically changed the wording of the corresponding DSM-III-R criterion to remove the requirement of a childhood history of Conduct Disorder.

(1) (Before the age of 15) often bullied, threatened, or intimidated others

> *Interviewer's Questions:* You've said that before you were 15, you would *[Before you were 15, would you]* bully or threaten other kids. Tell me about that.

Commentary: The implied threat must be of physical harm and not simply withdrawal of friendship.

(2) (Before the age of 15) often initiated physical fights

> *Interviewer's Questions:* You've said that before you were 15, you would *[Before you were 15, would you]* start fights. How often?

Commentary: This item should be rated "3" only if there is evidence that the person started fights, rather than just being drawn into them.

(3) (Before the age of 15) used a weapon that can cause serious physical harm to others (e.g., a bat, brick, broken bottle, knife, gun)

> *Interviewer's Questions:* You've said that before you were 15, you hurt or threatened someone *[Before you were 15, did you hurt or threaten someone]* with a weapon, like a bat, brick, broken bottle, knife, or gun. Tell me about that.

Commentary: Any use of a weapon warrants a rating of "3"—ranging from using a weapon in a fight to using a weapon to threaten, intimidate, rob, or sexually assault someone.

(4) (Before the age of 15) was physically cruel to people

> *Interviewer's Questions:* You've said that before you were 15, you deliberately tortured someone or caused someone physical pain and suffering. *[Before you were 15, did you deliberately torture someone or cause someone physical pain and suffering?]* What did you do?

Commentary: This refers to torturing or inflicting pain and suffering on others, apart from injuries inflicted during a fight. It also may include situations in which no actual physical pain is inflicted (e.g., locking a child in a closet).

(5) (Before the age of 15) was physically cruel to animals

> *Interviewer's Questions:* You've said that before you were 15 you tortured or hurt animals on purpose. *[Before you were 15, did you torture or hurt animals on purpose?]* What did you do?

Commentary: Being "physically cruel" implies purposely inflicting pain and suffering on the animal.

(6) (Before the age of 15) stole while confronting a victim (e.g., mugging, purse snatching, extortion, armed robbery)

> *Interviewer's Questions:* You've said that before you were 15, you robbed, mugged, or forcibly took *[Before you were 15, did you rob, mug, or forcibly take]* something from someone by threatening him or her. Tell me about that.

Commentary: This item requires face-to-face confrontation, ranging from verbal threats to actual violence.

(7) (Before the age of 15) forced someone into sexual activity

> *Interviewer's Questions:* You've said that before you were 15, you forced someone *[Before you were 15, did you force someone]* to have sex with you, to get undressed in front of you, or to touch you sexually. Tell me about it.

Commentary: This item refers to any coerced sexual activity, including rape, forcing someone to touch the person sexually, forcing someone to undress, or forcing someone to watch a sexual act.

(8) (Before the age of 15) deliberately engaged in fire setting with the intention of causing serious damage

> *Interviewer's Questions:* You've said that before you were 15 you *[Before you were 15, did you]* set fires. Tell me about that.

Commentary: The critical element is the intention, rather than whether or not the fire actually caused severe damage.

(9) (Before the age of 15) deliberately destroyed others' property (other than by fire setting)

> *Interviewer's Questions:* You've said that before you were 15, you deliberately destroyed *[Before you were 15, did you deliberately destroy]* things that weren't yours. What did you do?

Commentary: This item refers to vandalism of property with the intent to destroy, rather than purely as a form of expression (i.e., writing graffiti on a wall would not qualify, but breaking windows, trashing a house, putting dirt in a gas tank, or slashing tires would). Fire setting is excluded from this item because it is covered in the previous item.

(10) (Before the age of 15) broke into someone else's house, building, or car

> *Interviewer's Questions:* You've said that before you were 15, you broke *[Before you were 15,*

did you break] into houses, other buildings, or cars. Tell me about that.

(11) (Before the age of 15) often lied to obtain goods or favors or to avoid obligations (i.e., "cons" others)

Interviewer's Questions: You've said that before you were 15, you lied a lot or "conned" *[Before you were 15, did you lie a lot or "con"]* other people. What would you lie about?

Commentary: This question refers to manipulative lying. It does not include lying for other reasons, such as to avoid harsh punishment, get someone else in trouble, or keep one's parents at a distance.

(12) (Before the age of 15) stole items of nontrivial value without confronting a victim (e.g., shoplifting, stealing but without breaking and entering, forgery)

Interviewer's Questions: You've said that before you were 15, you sometimes stole or shoplifted things or forged someone's signature. *[Before you were 15, did you sometimes steal or shoplift things or forge someone's signature?]* Tell me about it.

Commentary: This item does not address stealing of trivial items (e.g., candy) or forging a signature for purposes other than theft.

(13) (Before the age of 15) ran away from home overnight at least twice while living in parental or parental surrogate home (or once without returning for a lengthy period)

Interviewer's Questions: You've said that before you were 15, you ran away from home and stayed *[Before you were 15, did you run away and stay]* away overnight. Was that more than once? (With whom were you living at the time?)

(14) (Before the age of 13) often stayed out at night despite parental prohibitions

Interviewer's Questions: You've said that before you were 13, you would *[Before you were 13, did you]* often stay out very late, long after the time you were supposed to be home. How often?

(15) (Before the age of 13) often truant from school
Interviewer's Questions: You've said that before you were 13, you often skipped *[Before you were 13, did you often skip]* school. How often?

Criterion A

(1) failure to conform to social norms with respect to lawful behaviors, as indicated by repeatedly performing acts that are grounds for arrest

Interviewer's Questions: Have you done things that are against the law—even if you weren't caught—like stealing, using or selling drugs, writing bad checks, or having sex for money? IF NO: Have you ever been arrested for anything?

Commentary: Note that this item refers to the social norms of the society at large (as defined by existing laws), as opposed to a subgroup that may condone certain illegal behavior. The acts, however, must be antisocial in nature—not acts of civil disobedience (e.g., trespassing while protesting).

(2) deceitfulness, as indicated by repeated lying, use of aliases, or "conning" others for personal profit or pleasure

Interviewer's Questions: Do you often find that you have to lie to get what you want? (Have you ever used an alias or pretended you were someone else?) (Have you often "conned" others to get what you want?)

Commentary: Individuals with this trait have no regard for the truth and lie to exploit others or maintain control over them. This item does not encompass lying to protect the person from harm (e.g., from spousal abuse).

(3) impulsivity or failure to plan ahead

Interviewer's Questions: Do you often do things on the spur of the moment without thinking about how it will affect you or other people? What kinds of things? Was there ever a time when you had no regular place to live? (For how long?)

Commentary: This trait involves making important decisions without any forethought or consideration of the implications to self or others. Examples include traveling from place to place without a prearranged job or adequate finances or the lack of a fixed address for a prolonged period of time. Note that a rating of "3" requires that the lack of planning be clearly irresponsible, not merely evidence of spontaneity.

(4) irritability and aggressiveness, as indicated by repeated physical fights or assaults

Interviewer's Questions: (Since you were 15) have you been in any fights? (How often?) Have you ever hit or thrown things at your spouse or partner? (How often?) Have you ever hit a child—yours or someone else's—so hard that he or she had bruises or had to stay in bed or see a doctor? Tell me about that. Have you physically threatened or hurt anyone else? Tell me about that. (How often?)

Commentary: Aggressive acts that are required to defend oneself or someone else or acts that are required by the person's job are not included as evidence for this trait.

(5) reckless disregard for safety of self or others

Interviewer's Questions: Did you ever drive a car when you were drunk or high? How many speeding tickets have you gotten or car accidents have you been in? Do you always use protection if you have sex with someone you don't know well? (Has anyone ever said that you allowed a child that you were taking care of to be in a dangerous situation?)

Commentary: This item includes situations in which the person ignores the safety of others. For example, the person may be so neglectful when caring for a child that the child gets into dangerous situations (e.g., allowing a child to wander onto a highway).

(6) consistent irresponsibility, as indicated by repeated failure to sustain consistent work behavior or honor financial obligations

Interviewer's Questions: How much of the time in the last 5 years were you not working? IF FOR A PROLONGED PERIOD: Why? (Was there work available?) When you were working, did you miss a lot of work? IF YES: Why? Did you ever walk off a job without having another one to go to? IF YES: How many times did this happen? Have you ever owed people money and not paid them back? (How often?) What about not paying child support, or not giving money to children or someone else who depended on you?

Commentary: There must be evidence of either irresponsible work behavior or financially irresponsibility. Irresponsible work behavior may be indicated by significant periods of unemployment despite available job opportunities, abandonment of several jobs without a realistic plan for getting another job, or repeated absences from work not explained by illness. Financial irresponsibility may be indicated by repeatedly defaulting on debts, refusal to pay child support or alimony, or repeated squandering on personal items of money required for household food or other necessities.

(7) lacks remorse, as indicated by being indifferent to or rationalizing having hurt, mistreated, or stolen from another

Interviewer's Questions: IF THERE IS EVIDENCE OF ANTISOCIAL ACTS AND IT IS

UNCLEAR WHETHER THERE IS ANY REMORSE: How do you feel about [LIST ANTISOCIAL ACTS]? (Do you think what you did was wrong in any way?)

Commentary: People with this trait lack any remorse about the consequences of their antisocial acts, often blaming the victims as being foolish, helpless, or deserving of their fate, or else minimizing the harmful consequences.

6. Training

Ideally, training should involve the following sequence:

1. Study the SCID-II User's Guide, familiarizing yourself with the basic features and conventions.

2. Carefully read through every word of SCID-II, making sure that you understand all of the instructions, questions, and diagnostic criteria. As you are reading through each criterion, refer to the corresponding item-by-item commentary.

3. Now practice reading the SCID-II questions aloud so that eventually SCID sounds as if it were your native tongue.

4. Watch the SCID-II videotape. Videotapes are available from Biometrics Research; call 212-960-5524.

When using the SCID-II in a research study with more than one interviewer, the following steps are recommended:

5. Try out SCID-II with a colleague (or significant other) who can assume the role of a subject.

6. Try out SCID-II on actual subjects who are as representative as possible of those who will be included in your research study. If possible, these rehearsals should be joint interviews, with all raters making independent ratings, followed by a discussion of the interviewing technique and all sources of disagreement in the ratings.

7. If possible, do a test-retest reliability study in which the interview is repeated with the same subject within a short period of time by a second interviewer. You will learn more from such a study if you audiotape the interviews, then have each interviewer listen to and rate the audiotape of the other interviewer, followed by a discussion of sources of disagreement.

   A test-retest reliability study may be impractical for some investigators. A less rigorous procedure for assessing the reliability of interviewers is to make a series of audio- or videotapes. In general, we would recommend a minimum of 10 joint interviews, although more would be better.

8. Investigators who are planning studies may wish to contact us about conducting a training workshop at your site (which would focus on direct supervision of live interviews) or reviewing a series of taped interviews made by your interviewers.

7. Data Processing

SCID-II does not require the use of a computer program to make the final DSM-IV diagnoses. However, to facilitate statistical analysis by computer and facilitate comparison of data between studies, the Scoresheet, the body of the SCID-II interview, and the Personality Questionnaire all have data field numbers on the right-hand side of each page. For most studies, data analysis will be confined to the Scoresheet. Other studies that are interested in the specific ratings made for the diagnostic criteria will need to utilize the fields from the body of the SCID-II itself.

We have also developed computer software to help administer SCID-II. Computer-Assisted SCID-II (CAS-II) is a Windows®-based computerized version of SCID-II developed by the authors in conjunction with Multi-Health Systems, a publisher and distributor of professional assessment and practice materials. The interviewer uses the CAS-II to administer the SCID-II interview in lieu of the paper version. It also integrates the item-by-item commentary contained in the User's Guide into the SCID-II interview, providing the user with the option of displaying the relevant commentary for each item. CAS-II also includes the SCID-II Patient Questionnaire (SCID-II-PQ), a computer-administered version of the Personality Questionnaire. SCID-II-PQ can be used as a stand-alone screener for personality disorders, or its results can be integrated with the CAS-II software so that questions answered "no" on the SCID-II-PQ cause the corresponding SCID-II criteria to be skipped during the interview. Call 1-800-456-3003 for more information about these products and ordering details.

8. Reliability and Validity

No data are available on the reliability or validity of the DSM-IV SCID-II, although a number of studies have been carried out that have investigated the reliability of its predecessor, the DSM-III-R SCID-II. We conducted a test-retest reliability study of the DSM-III-R SCID-II as part of a multisite reliability study of the SCID for Axis I Disorders (Williams et al. 1992). SCID-II interviews were administered by two separate interviewers on two different occasions (within 2 weeks) to 284 subjects in four psychiatric patient and two nonpsychiatric patient sites (First et al. 1995). For the patient sites, kappas ranged from .24 for Obsessive-Compulsive Personality Disorder to .74 for Histrionic Personality Disorder, with an overall weighted kappa of .53. For the nonpatients, however, agreement was considerably lower, with an overall weighted kappa of .38. Mean duration of administration time was 36 minutes.

The reliabilities obtained by other investigators using the SCID-II have varied widely but have actually equaled or exceeded the reliabilities in this study. Malow and colleagues (1989), after administering only the SCID-II sections for Borderline and Antisocial Personality Disorders, reported reliability on 29 cases selected from a larger sample of inpatients with either Cocaine or Opioid Dependence. Using a test-retest design (with the second interview occurring 48 hours after the first), they reported a kappa of .87 for Borderline Personality Disorder (base rate 16%) and .84 for Antisocial Personality Disorder (base rate 15%). O'Boyle and Self (1990) also reported test-retest reliability (mean time between interviews = 1.7 days) using the SCID-II on a sample of 18 inpatients. They calculated a kappa of .74 for the presence of any personality disorder (base rate of at least one personality disorder was 55%). Weiss and colleagues (1995) studied 12-month test-retest reliability on 31 cocaine-dependent patients and reported an overall kappa of .46.

Using a joint-reliability design, with one interviewer administering the SCID-II and the second interviewer acting as an observer, Arntz and colleagues (1992) investigated the reliability of a Dutch version of the SCID-II on a sample of 70 outpatients. For those disorders with at least five cases rated by either interviewer, kappas ranged from .77 for Obsessive-Compulsive Personality Disorder to .82 for Avoidant Personality Disorder; weighted kappa computed for all personality disorders was .80.

Four other studies employed a variant of the joint-reliability design, with the second interviewer making ratings using audiotapes (or videotapes) of the first interviewer as data. Renneberg and colleagues (1992) studied personality disorders in 32 anxious outpatients, reporting kappas of .75 for agreement on the presence of any personality disorder and kappas for individual disorders ranging from .61 for Paranoid Personality Disorder to .81 for Avoidant Personality Disorder. In a similarly designed study of personality disorders in patients with eating disorders, Wonderlich and colleagues (1990) reported SCID-II kappas ranging from .56 for Avoidant Personality Disorder to .77 for Obsessive-Compulsive Personality Disorder. Brooks and colleagues (1991) administered the SCID-II to 30 patients with Panic Disorder and Agoraphobia and reported kappas ranging from .43 for Histrionic Personality Disorder to .89 for Schizotypal Personality Disorder. Fogelson and colleagues (1991) rated personality disorders in a nonpatient sample of 45 first-degree relatives of patients with Schizophrenia, Schizoaffective Disorder, or Bipolar Disorder and reported intraclass correlation coefficients ranging from .60 for Schizoid Personality Disorder to .82 for Borderline Personality Disorder. These results obtained by us and by other investigators using the SCID-II underscore the variability of reliability in different settings, a finding that also applies to the reliability of Axis I disorders with structured diagnostic interviews. Overall, the results with the DSM-III-R SCID-II demonstrate that reasonable reliability can be obtained, provided that the interviewers are well-trained and that there is sufficient diagnostic variability in the sample.

Validity of the SCID-II has been investigated in several ways. Concurrent validity was demonstrated by Hueston and colleagues (1996) in a study that showed that in a group of primary care patients, having a personality disorder diagnosed by the SCID-II was associated with lower functional status, lower satisfaction with health care, and higher risk for depression and alcohol abuse. Most studies comparing the SCID-II to other personality measures are difficult to interpret because of a lack of a "gold" standard. For example, Hyler and colleagues (1992) demonstrated kappa agreements between the SCID-II and the Personality Disorder Examination (Loranger et al. 1987) ranging from .20 to .55 (mean .36) and agreements between the PDQ-R (a self-report questionnaire) and the SCID-II ranging from .02 to .53 (mean .38). Kennedy and colleagues (1995), however, demonstrated poor agreement between the SCID-II and the Millon Clinical Multiaxial Inventory (MCMI), another self-report instrument for assessing personality disorders.

A study by Skodol and colleagues (1991) compared the SCID-II and the Personality Disorder Examination (Loranger et al. 1987) and examined their agreement with each other and with a clinical standard (i.e., a longitudinal assessment procedure, given the acronym of the LEAD standard, for Longitudinal Expert evaluation using All Data [Spitzer 1983]). The study found only modest agreement between the two interviews, with the SCID-II slightly more valid than the Personality Disorder Examination compared with the clinical standard (i.e., the SCID-II had better agreement, as indicated by kappa, and better total predictive value, for 8 of the 11 personality disorders). The authors of the study conjecture that the greater agreement between the SCID-II and the LEAD standard may reflect either the greater similarity in the formats of these procedures (i.e., the criteria are evaluated disorder by disorder) or inherent advantages of the SCID, or both.

The validity of the SCID-II Personality Questionnaire was examined by Jacobsberg and colleagues (1995) by determining its false-positive rate using the Personality Disorder Examination as the standard. They found that the false-negative rate was low for every diagnosis and concluded that the SCID-II procedure of following up on positive responses was a valid method. Good agreement between the questionnaire and the SCID-II was demonstrated by Ekselius and colleagues (1994), demonstrating a correlation of .04 in the number of positive items and a kappa of .78.

9. References

American Psychiatric Association: Diagnostic and Statistical Manual of Mental Disorders, 4th Edition. Washington, DC, American Psychiatric Association, 1994

Arntz A, van Beijsterveldt B, Hoekstra R, et al: The interrater reliability of a Dutch version of the Structured Clinical Interview for DSM-III-R Personality Disorders. Acta Psychiatr Scand 85:394–400, 1992

Brooks RB, Baltazar PL, McDowell DE, et al: Personality disorders co-occurring with panic disorder with agoraphobia. Journal of Personality Disorders 5:327–336, 1991

Ekselius L, Lindstrom E, Von Knorring L, et al: SCID-II interviews and the SCID Screen Questionnaire as diagnostic tools for personality disorders in DSM-III-R. Acta Psychiatr Scand 90:120–123, 1994

First MB, Spitzer RL, Gibbon M, et al: The Structured Clinical Interview for DSM-III-R Personality Disorders (SCID-II), II: multi-site test-retest reliability study. Journal of Personality Disorders 9:92–104, 1995

Fogelson DL, Neuchterlein KH, Asarnow RF, et al: Interrater reliability of the Structured Clinical Interview for DSM-III-R, Axis II: schizophrenia spectrum and affective spectrum disorders. Psychiatry Res 39:55–63, 1991

Friedman CJ, Shear MK, Frances A: DSM-III personality disorders in panic patients. Journal of Personality Disorders 1:132–135, 1987

Green MA, Curtis GC: Personality disorders in panic patients: response to termination of antipanic medication. Journal of Personality Disorders 2:303–314, 1988

Hueston WJ, Mainous AG, Schilling R: Patients with personality disorders: functional status, health care utilization, and satisfaction with care. J Fam Pract 42:54–60, 1996

Hyler SE, Skodol AE, Oldham JM, et al: Validity of the Personality Disorder Questionnaire—Revised: a replication in an outpatient sample. Compr Psychiatry 33:734–737, 1992

Jacobsberg L, Perry S, Frances A: Diagnostic agreement between the SCID-II screening questionnaire and the Personality Disorder Examination. Journal of Personality Disorder Assessment 65:428–433, 1995

Kennedy SH, Katz R, Rockert W, et al: Assessment of personality disorders in anorexia nervosa and bulimia nervosa: a comparison of self-report and structured interview methods. J Nerv Ment Dis 193:358–364, 1995

Lofgren DP, Bemporad J, King J, et al: A prospective follow-up study of so-called borderline children. Am J Psychiatry 148:1541–1547, 1991

Loranger AW, Susman VL, Oldham JM, et al: The Personality Disorder Examination: a preliminary report. Journal of Personality Disorders 1:1–13, 1987

Malow RM, West JA, Williams JL, et al: Personality disorders classifications and symptoms in cocaine and opioid addicts. J Consult Clin Psychol 57:765–767, 1989

O'Boyle M, Self D: A comparison of two interviews for DSM-III-R personality disorders. Psychiatry Res 32:85–92, 1990

Renneberg B, Chambless DL, Dowdall DJ, et al: A structured interview for DSM-III-R, Axis II, and the Millon Clinical Multiaxial Inventory: a concurrent validity study of personality disorders among anxious outpatients. Journal of Personality Disorders 6:117–124, 1992

Schotte C, De Doncker D, Maes M, et al: Low MMPI diagnostic performance for the DSM-III-R obsessive-compulsive personality disorder. Psychol Rep 69:795–800, 1991a

Schotte C, Maes M, Cluydts R et al: MMPI characteristics of the DSM-III-R avoidant personality disorder. Psychol Rep 69:75–81, 1991b

Skodol AE, Oldham JM, Rosnick L, et al: Diagnosis of DSM-III-R personality disorders: a comparison of two structured interviews. International Journal of Methods in Psychiatric Research 1:13–26, 1991

Spitzer R: Psychiatric diagnosis: are clinicians still necessary? Compr Psychiatry 24:399–411, 1983

Weiss Rd, Najavits LM, Muenz LR, et al: Twelve-month test-retest reliability of the Structured Clinical Interview for DSM-III-R Personality Disorders in cocaine dependent patients. Compr Psychiatry 36:384–389, 1995

Williams JBW, Gibbon M, First MB, et al: The Structured Clinical Interview for DSM-III-R (SCID) II: multi-site test-retest reliability. Arch Gen Psychiatry 49:630–636, 1992

Wonderlich SA, Swift WJ, Slotnick HB, et al: DSM-III-R personality disorders in eating disorder subtypes. Int J Eat Disord 9:607–616, 1990

10. Appendix: Sample Case for SCID-II

During the course of a routine physical examination, Nick—a 25-year-old, single, African American man—unexpectedly starts crying and blurts out that he is very depressed and is thinking about a suicide attempt he made when he felt this way as a teenager. His doctor refers him for a psychiatric evaluation.

Nick is tall, bearded, muscular, and handsome. He is meticulously dressed in a white suit and has a rose in his lapel. He enters the psychiatrist's office, pauses dramatically, and exclaims, "Aren't roses wonderful this time of year?" When asked why he has come for an evaluation, Nick replies laughingly that he has done it to appease his family doctor, "who seemed worried about me." He also has read a book on psychotherapy and hopes that "maybe there is someone very special who can understand me. I'd make the most incredible patient." He then takes control of the interview and begins to talk about himself, after first remarking, half-jokingly, "I was hoping you would be as attractive as my family doctor."

Nick pulls from his attache case a series of newspaper clippings; his resume; photographs including some of himself with famous people; and a photocopied dollar bill with his face replacing George Washington's. Using these as cues, he begins to tell his story.

He explains that in the past few years he has "discovered" some now-famous actors, one of whom he describes as a "physically perfect teenage heartthrob." Nick volunteered to coordinate publicity for the actor; as part of that task, he posed in a bathing suit in a scene that resembled a famous scene from the actor's hit movie. Imitating the actor's voice, Nick laughingly, then seriously, describes how he and the actor had similar pasts: both were rejected by their parents and peers but overcame this rejection to become popular. When the actor came to town, Nick rented a limousine and showed up at the gala "as a joke," as though he were the star himself. The actor's agent expressed annoyance at what he had done, causing Nick to fly into a rage. When Nick cooled down, he realized that he was "wasting my time promoting others, and that it was time for me to start promoting myself." "Someday," he says, pointing to the picture of the actor, "he will want to be president of my fan club."

Although Nick has had little professional acting experience, he is sure that success is "only a question of time." He pulls out some promotional material he has written for his actors and says, "I should write letters to God—He'd love them!" When the psychiatrist is surprised that some materials are signed with a different name than the one Nick has given the receptionist, Nick pulls out a legal document explaining the name change. He has dropped his family name and taken as his second name his middle name.

When asked about his love life, Nick says he has no lover—and that this is because people are just "superficial." He then displays a newspaper clipping in which he had typeset his and his ex-lover's names in headlines that read: "The relationship is over." More recently he dated and adored a man with the same first name as his own; as he became disenchanted, however, he realized that the man was ugly and an embarrassment because he dressed so poorly. Nick then explains that he owns more than 100 neckties and about 30 suits and is proud of how much he spends on "putting myself together." He has no relationships with other homosexual men now, describing them as "only interested in sex." He considers heterosexual men to be "mindless and without aesthetic sense." The only people who have understood him are older men who have suffered as much as he has. "One day, the mindless, happy people who have ignored me will be lining up to see my movies."

Nick's father was very critical, an alcoholic who was rarely around and had many affairs. His

---

From Spitzer RL, Gibbon M, Skodol AE, Williams JBW, First MB: *DSM-IV Casebook.* Washington, DC, American Psychiatric Press, 1994, pp. 84–85. Used with permission.

mother was "like a friend." She was chronically depressed about her husband's affairs and turned to her son, often kissing him good night, until he was 18, when she started an affair of her own. Nick then felt abandoned and made his suicide gesture. He describes a tortured childhood, including being picked on by his peers for looking odd, until he began bodybuilding.

At the end of the interview, Nick is referred to an experienced clinician associated with the clinic, who charges a minimal fee ($10), which he can afford. However, Nick requests a referral to someone who would offer him free treatment, seeing no reason for paying anyone because the therapist "would be getting as much out of it as [he] would."

Discussion

Note that the questions whose numbers are circled on SCID-II correspond to the "yes" answers on the SCID-II Personality Questionnaire. Because the SCID-II interview focuses primarily on these circled questions, in most cases SCID-II items corresponding to questions that were not circled are left without a rating (indicating that these items were not explored during the interview). When following up on circled questions, the clinician should make a note of the content of the subject's response below the item to allow for a review of the evidence for making the ratings.

Throughout SCID-II, many items that the subject endorses on the Personality Questionnaire eventually end up with a rating of "1" or "2," generally because the subject misinterprets the intended meaning of the question or is unable to give sufficient evidence to support a rating of "3." For example, on page 2 of the SCID-II Personality Questionnaire, Nick answered "yes" to screening question 19 ("Do you have very high standards about what is right and what is wrong?") because he has very high standards about style and fashion. The question actually inquires, however, about the obsessive-compulsive trait of overconscientiousness and inflexibility about matters of morality, ethics, and values; thus this item (Obsessive-Compulsive Personality Disorder criterion 4, page 9) is rated "1." Similarly, the subject endorsed question 14 on page 2 of the SCID-II Personality Questionnaire ("When a close relationship ends, do you feel you immediately have to find someone else to take care of you?") because he went home to his mother after one breakup. Because this happened only on one occasion, the item (Dependent Personality Disorder criterion 7, page 7) is rated "2."

In the evaluation of Narcissistic Personality Disorder (pages 25–28), ratings are made for all of the items, even though the subject did not endorse all of the corresponding items on the Personality Questionnaire. Items originally answered negatively were explored a second time because the interviewer had the clinical impression that the patient exhibited narcissistic features. Similarly, after inquiring about the "yes" answers on the questionnaire, the interviewer was only one item short of making a diagnosis of Borderline Personality Disorder (items 1, 2, 4, and 6 were coded "3"; five items are required); all of the "no" answers for the remaining Borderline Personality Disorder items were reconfirmed during the SCID-II interview.

On the scoresheet, the subject is rated as having two personality disorders—namely Narcissistic Personality Disorder and Histrionic Personality Disorder, with seven items and five items respectively. Borderline Personality Disorder is rated as subthreshold because four of the nine items were coded "3" (five items coded "3" are required) and one item is coded "2."

STRUCTURED CLINICAL INTERVIEW
FOR DSM-IV AXIS II PERSONALITY DISORDERS

S C I D - II

Michael B. First, M.D.
Miriam Gibbon, M.S.W.
Robert L. Spitzer, M.D.
Janet B. W. Williams, D.S.W.

Biometrics Research Department
New York State Psychiatric Institute
Department of Psychiatry
Columbia University
New York, New York

Lorna Smith Benjamin, Ph.D.

Department of Psychology
University of Utah
Salt Lake City, Utah

Study: Clinic Intake Study No.: ___ ___ ___ ___ 1

Subject: Nick ID No.: 1 0 2 3 2

Interviewer: Gibbon Interviewer No.: ___ ___ ___ 3

Date of interview: 07 21 96 (Month Day Year) 4

Sources of information (check all that apply):

- [x] Subject 5
- [ ] Family/friends/associates 6
- [ ] Health professional/chart/referral note 7
- [x] SCID-II Personality Questionnaire 8

Edited and checked by: First Date: 7/25/96

SCID-II SUMMARY SCORESHEET

Overall quality and completeness of information:

1 = poor, 2 = fair, (3) = good, 4 = excellent 9

Duration of interview (minutes) 0 3 0 10

Personality Disorder

Number of Items Coded "3"
(Boxed numbers indicate threshold required for a diagnosis.)

01	Avoidant *(pp. 3–4)*	1	2	3	[4]	5	6	7			11
02	Dependent *(pp. 5–7)*	1	2	3	4	[5]	6	7	8		12
03	Obsessive-Compulsive *(pp. 8–10)*	(1)	2	3	[4]	5	6	7	8		13
04	Passive-Aggressive *(pp. 11–12)*	1	2	3	[4]	5	6	7			14
05	Depressive *(pp. 13–14)*	1	2	3	4	[5]	6	7			15
06	Paranoid *(pp. 15–16)*	1	2	3	[4]	5	6	7			16
07	Schizotypal *(pp. 17–20)*	1	2	3	4	[5]	6	7	8	9	17
08	Schizoid *(pp. 21–22)*	1	2	3	[4]	5	6	7			18
09	Histrionic *(pp. 23–24)*	1	2	3	4	([5])	6	7	8		19
10	Narcissistic *(pp. 25–28)*	1	2	3	4	[5]	6	(7)	8	9	20
11	Borderline *(pp. 29–32)*	1	2	3	(4)	[5]	6	7	8	9	21
12	Antisocial *(pp. 33–40)*	1	2	[3]	4	5	6	7			22
13	Not Otherwise Specified (NOS) *(p. 41)*	[1]									23

PRINCIPAL AXIS II DIAGNOSIS (i.e., the Personality Disorder that is—or should be—the main focus of clinical attention).

Enter code number from left of diagnosis above: 1 0 24
Note: Enter 99 if no Axis II disorder.

OVERVIEW FOR PERSONALITY DISORDERS

Now I am going to ask you some questions about the kind of person you are—that is, how you generally have felt or behaved.

IF A CIRCUMSCRIBED OR EPISODIC AXIS I DISORDER HAS BEEN PRESENT: I know that there have been times when you have been [AXIS I SYMPTOMS]. I am not talking about those times; you should try to think of how you *usually* are when you are not [AXIS I SYMPTOMS]. Do you have any questions about this?

How would you describe yourself as a person (before [AXIS I SYMPTOMS])?

talented, handsome

IF CAN'T ANSWER, MOVE ON.

How do you think other people would describe you as a person (before [AXIS I SYMPTOMS])?

friendly, loving

Who have been the important people in your life?

mother — some friends & lovers

(IF MENTIONS ONLY FAMILY: What about friends?)

How have you gotten along with them?

OK

Do you think that the usual way that you react to things or behave with people has caused you problems with anyone? (At home? At school? At work?) (In what way?)

No

What kinds of things have you done that other people might have found annoying?

Sometimes I'm too hones-

How do you spend your free time?

acting classes, fan club

If you could change your personality in some ways, how would you want to be different?

more decisive

→ IF PERSONALITY QUESTIONNAIRE HAS BEEN COMPLETED: Now I want to go over the questions to which you answered "yes" on the questionnaire.

→ IF PERSONALITY QUESTIONNAIRE HAS NOT BEEN COMPLETED: Now I want to ask you some more specific questions.

SCID-II

PERSONALITY QUESTIONNAIRE

(To be used with SCID-II Interview)

Your initials: N A K

Today's date: 07 21 96 PQ1

Month Day Year

Study No.: __ __ __ __ PQ2

ID No.: 1 0 2 3 PQ3

(to be completed by study staff)

Instructions

These questions are about the kind of person you generally are—that is, how you have usually felt or behaved over the past several years. Circle "YES" if the question completely or mostly applies to you, or circle "NO" if it does not apply to you. If you do not understand a question or are not sure of your answer, leave it blank.

1.	Have you avoided jobs or tasks that involved having to deal with a lot of people?	NO	YES	PQ4
2.	Do you avoid getting involved with people unless you are certain they will like you?	NO	YES	PQ5
3.	Do you find it hard to be "open" even with people you are close to?	NO	YES	PQ6
4.	Do you often worry about being criticized or rejected in social situations?	NO	YES	PQ7
5.	Are you usually quiet when you meet new people?	NO	YES	PQ8
6.	Do you believe that you're not as good, as smart, or as attractive as most other people?	NO	YES	PQ9
7.	Are you afraid to try new things?	NO	YES	PQ10
8.	Do you need a lot of advice or reassurance from others before you can make everyday decisions—like what to wear or what to order in a restaurant?	NO	YES	PQ11
9.	Do you depend on other people to handle important areas in your life such as finances, child care, or living arrangements?	NO	YES	PQ12
10.	Do you find it hard to disagree with people even when you think they are wrong?	NO	YES	PQ13
11.	Do you find it hard to start or work on tasks when there is no one to help you?	NO	YES	PQ14
12.	Have you often volunteered to do things that are unpleasant?	NO	YES	PQ15
13.	Do you usually feel uncomfortable when you are by yourself?	NO	YES	PQ16

14. When a close relationship ends, do you feel you immediately have to find someone else to take care of you?	NO	**YES**	PQ17
15. Do you worry a lot about being left alone to take care of yourself?	**NO**	YES	PQ18
16. Are you the kind of person who focuses on details, order, and organization or likes to make lists and schedules?	**NO**	YES	PQ19
17. Do you have trouble finishing jobs because you spend so much time trying to get things exactly right?	**NO**	YES	PQ20
18. Do you or other people feel that you are so devoted to work (or school) that you have no time left for anyone else or for just having fun?	**NO**	YES	PQ21
19. Do you have very high standards about what is right and what is wrong?	NO	**YES**	PQ22
20. Do you have trouble throwing things out because they might come in handy some day?	**NO**	YES	PQ23
21. Is it hard for you to let other people help you unless they agree to do things exactly the way you want?	NO	**YES**	PQ24
22. Is it hard for you to spend money on yourself and other people even when you have enough?	**NO**	YES	PQ25
23. Are you often so sure you are right that it doesn't matter what other people say?	NO	**YES**	PQ26
24. Have other people told you that you are stubborn or rigid?	**NO**	YES	PQ27
25. When someone asks you to do something that you don't want to do, do you say "yes" but then work slowly or do a bad job?	**NO**	YES	PQ28
26. If you don't want to do something, do you often just "forget" to do it?	NO	**YES**	PQ29
27. Do you often feel that other people don't understand you, or don't appreciate how much you do?	NO	**YES**	PQ30
28. Are you often grumpy and likely to get into arguments?	**NO**	YES	PQ31

29. Have you found that most of your bosses, teachers, supervisors, doctors, and others who are supposed to know what they are doing really don't?	NO	YES	PQ32
30. Do you often think that it's not fair that other people have more than you do?	NO	YES	PQ33
31. Do you often complain that more than your share of bad things have happened to you?	NO	YES	PQ34
32. Do you often angrily refuse to do what others want and then later feel bad and apologize?	NO	YES	PQ35
33. Do you usually feel unhappy or that life is no fun?	NO	YES	PQ36
34. Do you believe that you are basically an inadequate person and often don't feel good about yourself?	NO	YES	PQ37
35. Do you often put yourself down?	NO	YES	PQ38
36. Do you keep thinking about bad things that have happened in the past or worry about bad things that might happen in the future?	NO	YES	PQ39
37. Do you often judge others harshly and easily find fault with them?	NO	YES	PQ40
38. Do you think that most people are basically no good?	NO	YES	PQ41
39. Do you almost always expect things to turn out badly?	NO	YES	PQ42
40. Do you often feel guilty about things you have or haven't done?	NO	YES	PQ43
41. Do you often have to keep an eye out to stop people from using you or hurting you?	NO	YES	PQ44
42. Do you spend a lot of time wondering if you can trust your friends or the people you work with?	NO	YES	PQ45
43. Do you find that it is best not to let other people know much about you because they will use it against you?	NO	YES	PQ46
44. Do you often detect hidden threats or insults in things people say or do?	NO	YES	PQ47

45. Are you the kind of person who holds grudges or takes a long time to forgive people who have insulted or slighted you?	(NO)	YES	PQ48
46. Are there many people you can't forgive because they did or said something to you a long time ago?	(NO)	YES	PQ49
47. Do you often get angry or lash out when someone criticizes or insults you in some way?	NO	(YES)	PQ50
48. Have you often suspected that your spouse or partner has been unfaithful?	NO	(YES)	PQ51
49. When you are out in public and see people talking, do you often feel that they are talking about you?	NO	(YES)	PQ52
50. Do you often get the feeling that things that have no special meaning to most people are really meant to give you a message?	(NO)	YES	PQ53
51. When you are around people, do you often get the feeling that you are being watched or stared at?	NO	(YES)	PQ54
52. Have you ever felt that you could make things happen just by making a wish or thinking about them?	(NO)	YES	PQ55
53. Have you had personal experiences with the supernatural?	(NO)	YES	PQ56
54. Do you believe that you have a "sixth sense" that allows you to know and predict things that others can't?	(NO)	YES	PQ57
55. Does it often seem that objects or shadows are really people or animals or that noises are actually people's voices?	(NO)	YES	PQ58
56. Have you had the sense that some person or force is around you, even though you cannot see anyone?	(NO)	YES	PQ59
57. Do you often see auras or energy fields around people?	(NO)	YES	PQ60
58. Are there very few people that you're really close to outside of your immediate family?	(NO)	YES	PQ61
59. Do you often feel nervous when you are with other people?	(NO)	YES	PQ62
60. Is it NOT important to you whether you have any close relationships?	(NO)	YES	PQ63

61.	Would you almost always rather do things alone than with other people?	**NO**	YES	PQ64
62.	Could you be content without ever being sexually involved with anyone?	**NO**	YES	PQ65
63.	Are there really very few things that give you pleasure?	**NO**	YES	PQ66
64.	Does it NOT matter to you what people think of you?	**NO**	YES	PQ67
65.	Do you find that nothing makes you very happy or very sad?	**NO**	YES	PQ68
66.	Do you like to be the center of attention?	NO	**YES**	PQ69
67.	Do you flirt a lot?	NO	**YES**	PQ70
68.	Do you often find yourself "coming on" to people?	**NO**	YES	PQ71
69.	Do you try to draw attention to yourself by the way you dress or look?	NO	**YES**	PQ72
70.	Do you often make a point of being dramatic and colorful?	NO	**YES**	PQ73
71.	Do you often change your mind about things depending on the people you're with or what you have just read or seen on TV?	**NO**	YES	PQ74
72.	Do you have lots of friends that you are very close to?	**NO**	YES	PQ75
73.	Do people often fail to appreciate your very special talents or accomplishments?	NO	**YES**	PQ76
74.	Have people told you that you have too high an opinion of yourself?	NO	**YES**	PQ77
75.	Do you think a lot about the power, fame, or recognition that will be yours someday?	NO	**YES**	PQ78
76.	Do you think a lot about the perfect romance that will be yours someday?	**NO**	YES	PQ79
77.	When you have a problem, do you almost always insist on seeing the top person?	NO	**YES**	PQ80

78. Do you feel it is important to spend time with people who are special or influential?	NO	YES	PQ81
79. Is it very important to you that people pay attention to you or admire you in some way?	NO	YES	PQ82
80. Do you think that it's not necessary to follow certain rules or social conventions when they get in your way?	NO	YES	PQ83
81. Do you feel that you are the kind of person who deserves special treatment?	NO	YES	PQ84
82. Do you often find it necessary to step on a few toes to get what you want?	NO	YES	PQ85
83. Do you often have to put your needs above other people's?	NO	YES	PQ86
84. Do you often expect other people to do what you ask without question because of who you are?	NO	YES	PQ87
85. Are you NOT really interested in other people's problems or feelings?	NO	YES	PQ88
86. Have people complained to you that you don't listen to them or care about their feelings?	NO	YES	PQ89
87. Are you often envious of others?	NO	YES	PQ90
88. Do you feel that others are often envious of you?	NO	YES	PQ91
89. Do you find that there are very few people that are worth your time and attention?	NO	YES	PQ92
90. Have you often become frantic when you thought that someone you really cared about was going to leave you?	NO	YES	PQ93
91. Do your relationships with people you really care about have lots of extreme ups and downs?	NO	YES	PQ94
92. Have you all of a sudden changed your sense of who you are and where you are headed?	NO	YES	PQ95
93. Does your sense of who you are often change dramatically?	NO	YES	PQ96

94. Are you different with different people or in different situations, so that you sometimes don't know who you really are?	**NO**	YES	PQ97
95. Have there been lots of sudden changes in your goals, career plans, religious beliefs, and so on?	**NO**	YES	PQ98
96. Have you often done things impulsively?	NO	**YES**	PQ99
97. Have you tried to hurt or kill yourself or threatened to do so?	NO	**YES**	PQ100
98. Have you ever cut, burned, or scratched yourself on purpose?	**NO**	YES	PQ101
99. Do you have a lot of sudden mood changes?	NO	**YES**	PQ102
100. Do you often feel empty inside?	**NO**	YES	PQ103
101. Do you often have temper outbursts or get so angry that you lose control?	**NO**	YES	PQ104
102. Do you hit people or throw things when you get angry?	**NO**	YES	PQ105
103. Do even little things get you very angry?	**NO**	YES	PQ106
104. When you are under a lot of stress, do you get suspicious of other people or feel especially spaced out?	**NO**	YES	PQ107
105. Before you were 15, would you bully or threaten other kids?	**NO**	YES	PQ108
106. Before you were 15, would you start fights?	**NO**	YES	PQ109
107. Before you were 15, did you hurt or threaten someone with a weapon, like a bat, brick, broken bottle, knife, or gun?	**NO**	YES	PQ110
108. Before you were 15, did you deliberately torture someone or cause someone physical pain and suffering?	**NO**	YES	PQ111
109. Before you were 15, did you torture or hurt animals on purpose?	**NO**	YES	PQ112
110. Before you were 15, did you rob, mug, or forcibly take something from someone by threatening him or her?	**NO**	YES	PQ113

111. Before you were 15, did you force someone to have sex with you, to get undressed in front of you, or to touch you sexually?	NO	YES	PQ114
112. Before you were 15, did you set fires?	NO	YES	PQ115
113. Before you were 15, did you deliberately destroy things that weren't yours?	NO	YES	PQ116
114. Before you were 15, did you break into houses, other buildings, or cars?	NO	YES	PQ117
115. Before you were 15, did you lie a lot or "con" other people?	NO	YES	PQ118
116. Before you were 15, did you sometimes steal or shoplift things or forge someone's signature?	NO	YES	PQ119
117. Before you were 15, did you run away from home and stay away overnight?	NO	YES	PQ120
118. Before you were 13, did you often stay out very late, long after the time you were supposed to be home?	NO	YES	PQ121
119. Before you were 13, did you often skip school?	NO	YES	PQ122

AVOIDANT PERSONALITY DISORDER	AVOIDANT PERSONALITY DISORDER CRITERIA		
	A pervasive pattern of social inhibition, feelings of inadequacy, and hypersensitivity to negative evaluation, beginning by early adulthood and present in a variety of contexts, as indicated by four (or more) of the following:		
1. You've said that you have *[Have you]* avoided jobs or tasks that involved having to deal with a lot of people. Give me some examples. What was the reason that you avoided these [LIST JOBS OR TASKS]? (Have you ever refused a promotion because it would involve dealing with more people than you would be comfortable with?)	(1) avoids occupational activities that involve significant interpersonal contact because of fears of criticism, disapproval, or rejection 3 = at least two examples	? 1 2 3	25
2. You've said that *[Do]* you avoid getting involved with people unless you are certain they will like you. If you don't know whether someone likes you, would you ever make the first move?	(2) is unwilling to get involved with people unless certain of being liked 3 = almost never takes the initiative in becoming involved in a social relationship	? 1 2 3	26
3. You've said that *[Do]* you find it hard to be "open" even with people you are close to. Why is this? (Are you afraid of being made fun of or embarrassed?)	(3) shows restraint within intimate relationships because of the fear of being shamed or ridiculed 3 = true for almost all relationships	? 1 2 3	27

? = inadequate information 1 = absent or false 2 = subthreshold 3 = threshold or true

4. You've said that *[Do]* you often worry about being criticized or rejected in social situations. Give me some examples. Do you spend a lot of time worrying about this?	(4) is preoccupied with being criticized or rejected in social situations 3 = a lot of time spent worrying about social situations	? 1 2 3	28
5. You've said that you're *[Are you]* usually quiet when you meet new people. Why is that? (Is it because you feel in some way inadequate, or not good enough?)	(5) is inhibited in new interpersonal situations because of feelings of inadequacy 3 = acknowledges trait and many examples	? 1 2 3	29
6. You've said that *[Do]* you believe that you're not as good, as smart, or as attractive as most other people. Tell me about that.	(6) views self as socially inept, personally unappealing, or inferior to others 3 = acknowledges belief	? 1 2 3	30
7. You've said that you're *[Are you]* afraid to try new things. Is that because you are afraid of being embarrassed? Give me some examples.	(7) is unusually reluctant to take personal risks or to engage in any new activities because they may prove embarrassing 3 = several examples of avoiding activities because of fear of embarrassment	? 1 2 3	31
	AT LEAST FOUR ITEMS ARE CODED "3"	1 3 ↓ **AVOIDANT PERSONALITY DISORDER**	32

? = inadequate information **1 = absent or false** **2 = subthreshold** **3 = threshold or true**

DEPENDENT PERSONALITY DISORDER

DEPENDENT PERSONALITY DISORDER CRITERIA

A pervasive and excessive need to be taken care of that leads to submissive and clinging behavior and fears of separation, beginning by early adulthood and present in a variety of contexts, as indicated by five (or more) of the following:

8. You've said that *[Do]* you need a lot of advice or reassurance from others before you can make everyday decisions—like what to wear or what to order in a restaurant.

Can you give me some examples of the kinds of decisions you would ask for advice or reassurance about?

(Does this happen most of the time?)

(1) has difficulty making everyday decisions without an excessive amount of advice and reassurance from others

3 = several examples

Sometimes — what to wear

? 1 2 3 33

9. You've said that you *[Do you]* depend on other people to handle important areas in your life such as finances, child care, or living arrangements.

Give me some examples. (Is this more than just getting advice from people?)

(Has this happened with MOST important areas of your life?)

(2) needs others to assume responsibility for most major areas of his or her life

[Note: Do not include merely getting advice from others or subculturally expected behavior.]

3 = several examples

? 1 2 3 34

? = inadequate information 1 = absent or false 2 = subthreshold 3 = threshold or true

10. You've said that *[Do]* you find it hard to disagree with people even when you think they are wrong. Give me some examples of when you've found it hard to disagree. What are you afraid will happen if you disagree?	(3) has difficulty expressing disagreement with others because of fear of loss of support or approval (**Note:** Do not include realistic fears of retribution.) 3 = acknowledges trait or several examples	? 1 2 3	35
11. You've said *[Do]* you find it hard to start or work on tasks when there is no one to help you. Give me some examples. Why is that? (Is this because you are not sure you can do it right?)	(4) has difficulty initiating projects or doing things on his or her own (because of a lack of self-confidence in judgment or abilities rather than a lack of motivation or energy) 3 = acknowledges trait	? 1 2 3	36
12. You've said that you have *[Have you]* often volunteered to do things that are unpleasant. Give me some examples of these kinds of things. Why is that?	(5) goes to excessive lengths to obtain nurturance and support from others, to the point of volunteering to do things that are unpleasant [Note: Do not include behavior intended to achieve goals other than being liked, such as job advancement.] 3 = acknowledges trait and at least one example	? 1 2 3	37
13. You've said that [*Do*] you usually feel uncomfortable when you are by yourself. Why is that? (Is it because you need someone to take care of you?)	(6) feels uncomfortable or helpless when alone, because of exaggerated fears of being unable to care for himself or herself 3 = acknowledges trait	? 1 2 3	38

? = inadequate information 1 = absent or false 2 = subthreshold 3 = threshold or true

Interview question	Criterion	Rating	Item
14. You've said that when a close relationship ends you *[When a close relationship ends, do you]* feel you immediately have to find someone else to take care of you. Tell me about that. (Have you reacted this way almost always when close relationships have ended?)	(7) urgently seeks another relationship as a source of care and support when a close relationship ends 3 = happens when most close relationships end with first lover— went home to live with mother	? 1 (2) 3	39
15. You've said that *[Do]* you worry a lot about being left alone to take care of yourself. Are there often times when you keep worrying about this? Do you have periods when you worry about this all the time?	(8) is unrealistically preoccupied with fears of being left to take care of himself or herself 3 = persistent unrealistic worry	? 1 2 3	40
	AT LEAST FIVE ITEMS ARE CODED "3"	(1) 3 ↓ **DEPENDENT PERSONALITY DISORDER**	41

? = inadequate information 1 = absent or false 2 = subthreshold 3 = threshold or true

OBSESSIVE-COMPULSIVE PERSONALITY DISORDER	OBSESSIVE-COMPULSIVE PERSONALITY DISORDER CRITERIA		
	A pervasive pattern of preoccupation with orderliness, perfectionism, and mental and interpersonal control, at the expense of flexibility, openness, and efficiency, beginning by early adulthood and present in a variety of contexts, as indicated by four (or more) of the following:		
16. You've said that you are *[Are you]* the kind of person who focuses on details, order, and organization or likes to make lists and schedules. Give me some examples. Do you sometimes get so caught up with [EXAMPLES] that you lose sight of what you are trying to accomplish? (. . . Like you can't see the forest for the trees?) (Does this happen often?)	(1) is preoccupied with details, rules, lists, order, organization, or schedules to the extent that the major point of the activity is lost 3 = acknowledges trait and at least one example	? 1 2 3	42
17. You've said that *[Do]* you have trouble finishing jobs because you spend so much time trying to get things exactly right. Give me some examples. (How often does this happen?)	(2) shows perfectionism that interferes with task completion (e.g., is unable to complete a project because his or her own overly strict standards are not met) 3 = several examples of tasks not completed or significantly delayed because of perfectionism	? 1 2 3	43

? = inadequate information 1 = absent or false 2 = subthreshold 3 = threshold or true

18. You've said that you or other people feel that you *[Do you or other people feel that you]* are so devoted to work (or school) that you have no time left for anyone else or for just having fun. Tell me about it.	(3) is excessively devoted to work and productivity to the exclusion of leisure activities and friendships (not accounted for by obvious economic necessity) [Note: Also not accounted for by temporary job requirements.] 3 = acknowledges trait or has been told by other people	? 1 2 3	44
19. You've said that *[Do]* you have very high standards about what is right and what is wrong. Give me some examples of your high standards. (Do you follow rules to the letter of the law, no matter what?) IF GIVES RELIGIOUS EXAMPLE: Do even people who share your religious views say you're too strict about right and wrong?	(4) is overconscientious, scrupulous, and inflexible about matters of morality, ethics, or values (not accounted for by cultural or religious identification) 3 = several examples of holding self or others to rigidly high moral standards about how I look and dress	? 1 2 3	45
20. You've said that *[Do]* you have trouble throwing things out because they might come in handy some day. Give me some examples of things that you're unable to throw out. (How cluttered does your place get because you don't throw things out?)	(5) is unable to discard worn-out or worthless objects even when they have no sentimental value 3 = results in a cluttered environment	? 1 2 3	46

? = inadequate information 1 = absent or false 2 = subthreshold 3 = threshold or true

21. You've said that it is *[Is it]* hard for you to let other people help you unless they agree to do things exactly the way you want. Tell me about that. (Does this happen often?) (Do you often end up doing things yourself to make sure they are done right?)	(6) is reluctant to delegate tasks or to work with others unless they submit to exactly his or her way of doing things 3 = acknowledges trait and at least one example want things to look just right. Example: dinner parties, have to do it all myself	? 1 2 3	47
22. You've said that it is *[Is it]* hard for you to spend money on yourself and other people even when you have enough. Why? (Is this because you're worried about not having enough in the future when you really need it?) Tell me about some things you haven't spent money on because you have to save for the future.	(7) adopts a miserly spending style toward both self and others; money is viewed as something to be hoarded for future catastrophes 3 = acknowledges trait and at least one example	? 1 2 3	48
23. You've said that you are *[Are you]* often so sure you are right that it doesn't matter what other people say. Tell me about it. 24. You've said that other people have told you *[Have other people told you]* that you are stubborn or rigid. Tell me about that.	(8) shows rigidity and stubbornness 3 = acknowledges trait or has been told by other people In matters of taste — I just have an eye for what looks good	? 1 2 3	49
	AT LEAST FOUR ITEMS ARE CODED "3"	1 3 → **OBSESSIVE-COMPULSIVE PERSONALITY DISORDER**	50

? = inadequate information 1 = absent or false 2 = subthreshold 3 = threshold or true

PASSIVE-AGGRESSIVE PERSONALITY DISORDER

PASSIVE-AGGRESSIVE PERSONALITY DISORDER CRITERIA

A pervasive pattern of negativistic attitudes and passive resistance to demands for adequate performance, beginning by early adulthood and present in a variety of contexts, as indicated by four (or more) of the following:

25. You've said that when someone asks you to do something that you don't want to do, you *[When someone asks you to do something that you don't want to do, do you]* say "yes" but then work slowly or do a bad job.

Give me some examples of this.

26. You've said that if you don't want to do something you *[If you don't want to do something, do you]* often just "forget" to do it.

Give me some examples of this.

(1) passively resists fulfilling routine social and occupational tasks ? 1 (2) 3 51

3 = acknowledges trait and at least one example

Sometimes it's easier to say you forgot
Example: didn't feel like going to gallery opening

27. You've said that *[Do]* you often feel that other people don't understand you or don't appreciate how much you do.

Tell me more about that. (Do you complain to other people about this?)

(2) complains of being misunderstood and unappreciated by others ? (1) 2 3 52

3 = acknowledges trait

people don't recognize how talented I am

28. You've said that you're *[Are you]* often grumpy and likely to get into arguments.

Tell me when this happens.

(3) is sullen and argumentative ? 1 2 3 53

3 = acknowledges trait

? = inadequate information 1 = absent or false 2 = subthreshold 3 = threshold or true

29. You've said that you've *[Have you]* found that most of your bosses, teachers, supervisors, doctors, and others who are supposed to know what they are doing really don't. Tell me about that.	(4) unreasonably criticizes and scorns authority 3 = several examples	? 1 2 3	54
30. You've said that *[Do]* you often think that it's not fair that other people have more than you do. Tell me more about that.	(5) expresses envy and resentment toward those apparently more fortunate 3 = examples of envy and resentment Some people don't deserve it — my time will come	? (1) 2 3	55
31. You've said that *[Do]* you often complain that more than your share of bad things have happened to you. Looking back on your life, do you feel that bad things are always happening to you?	(6) voices exaggerated and persistent complaints of personal misfortune 3 = says bad things always happen (not limited to particularly bad times in the person's life)	? 1 2 3	56
32. You've said that *[Do]* you often angrily refuse to do what others want and then later feel bad and apologize. Tell me more about this.	(7) alternates between hostile defiance and contrition 3 = acknowledges trait and at least one example	? 1 2 3	57
	AT LEAST FOUR ITEMS ARE CODED "3"	(1) 3 ↓ **PASSIVE-AGGRESSIVE PERSONALITY DISORDER**	58

? = inadequate information **1 = absent or false** **2 = subthreshold** **3 = threshold or true**

DEPRESSIVE PERSONALITY DISORDER	DEPRESSIVE PERSONALITY DISORDER CRITERIA		
Note: The DSM-IV criterion excludes a diagnosis of Depressive Personality Disorder if the behavior occurs only during Major Depressive Episodes or is better accounted for by Dysthymic Disorder. Refer to the User's Guide for a discussion of options for operationalizing this criterion.	A pervasive pattern of depressive cognitions and behaviors, beginning by early adulthood and present in a variety of contexts, as indicated by five (or more) of the following:		
33. You've said that *[Do]* you usually feel unhappy or that life is no fun. Tell me about that.	(1) usual mood is dominated by dejection, gloominess, cheerlessness, joylessness, unhappiness 3 = acknowledges trait	? 1 2 3	59
34. You've said that *[Do]* you believe that you are basically an inadequate person and often don't feel good about yourself. Tell me about that.	(2) self-concept centers around beliefs of inadequacy, worthlessness, and low self-esteem 3 = acknowledges trait	? 1 2 3	60
35. You've said that you *[Do you]* often put yourself down. Tell me about that. (Do you often blame yourself for things that haven't worked out?)	(3) is critical, blaming, and derogatory toward self 3 = acknowledges trait	? 1 2 3	61
36. You've said that *[Do]* you keep thinking about bad things that have happened in the past or worry about bad things that might happen in the future. Tell me about that.	(4) is brooding and given to worry 3 = acknowledges trait	? 1 2 3	62

? = inadequate information 1 = absent or false 2 = subthreshold 3 = threshold or true

37. You've said that *[Do]* you often judge others harshly and easily find fault with them. Give me some examples of the kinds of things you are critical of.	(5) is negativistic, critical, and judgmental toward others 3 = acknowledges trait and at least one example	? 1 2 3	63
38. You've said that you *[Do you]* think that most people are basically no good. Tell me about that.			
39. You've said that you *[Do you]* almost always expect things to turn out badly. Tell me about that.	(6) is pessimistic 3 = acknowledges trait	? 1 2 3	64
40. You've said that you *[Do you]* often feel guilty about things you have or haven't done. What kinds of things?	(7) is prone to feeling guilty or remorseful 3 = acknowledges trait and at least one example	? 1 2 3	65
	AT LEAST FIVE ITEMS ARE CODED "3"	(1) 3 ↓ **DEPRESSIVE PERSONALITY DISORDER**	66

? = inadequate information **1 = absent or false** **2 = subthreshold** **3 = threshold or true**

PARANOID PERSONALITY DISORDER	PARANOID PERSONALITY DISORDER CRITERIA		
Note: Behavior should NOT be considered characteristic of Paranoid Personality Disorder if it occurs exclusively during the course of Schizophrenia, a Mood Disorder With Psychotic Features, or another Psychotic Disorder or is due to the direct physiological effects of a general medical condition.	A pervasive distrust and suspiciousness of others such that their motives are interpreted as malevolent, beginning by early adulthood and present in a variety of contexts, as indicated by four (or more) of the following:		
41. You've said that *[Do]* you often have to keep an eye out to stop people from using you or hurting you. Tell me about that.	(1) suspects, without sufficient basis, that others are exploiting, harming, or deceiving him or her 3 = acknowledges trait and at least one example	? 1 2 3	67
42. You've said that you *[Do you]* spend a lot of time wondering if you can trust your friends or the people you work with. Describe situations where you've gotten that feeling. (Do you feel this way often?)	(2) is preoccupied with unjustified doubts about the loyalty or trustworthiness of friends or associates 3 = acknowledges that this is characteristic of almost all relationships not with friends— but have to be careful with showbiz types— everyone out for himself	? 1 (2) 3	68
43. You've said that *[Do]* you find that it is best not to let other people know much about you because they will use it against you. When has this happened? Tell me about it.	(3) is reluctant to confide in others because of unwarranted fear that the information will be used maliciously against him or her 3 = acknowledges that reluctance to confide in others is due to mistrust (not merely fear of rejection)	? 1 2 3	69
44. You've said that *[Do]* you often detect hidden threats or insults in things people say or do. Give me some examples.	(4) reads hidden demeaning or threatening meanings into benign remarks or events 3 = acknowledges trait and at least one example	? 1 2 3	70

? = inadequate information 1 = absent or false 2 = subthreshold 3 = threshold or true

Question	Criterion	Rating	Item
45. You've said that you're *[Are you]* the kind of person who holds grudges or takes a long time to forgive people who have insulted or slighted you. Tell me about that. 46. You've said that there are *[Are there]* many people you can't forgive because they did or said something to you a long time ago. Tell me about that.	(5) persistently bears grudges (i.e., is unforgiving of insults, injuries, or slights) 3 = acknowledges trait and at least one example	? 1 2 3	71
(47.) You've said that *[Do]* you often get angry or lash out when someone criticizes or insults you in some way. Give me some examples. (Do others believe that you often take offense too easily?)	(6) perceives attacks on his or her character or reputation that are not apparent to others and is quick to react angrily or to counterattack 3 = acknowledges trait and at least one example I have a temper— Example: really pissed when that agent told me to get out	? (1) 2 3	72
(48.) You've said that you have *[Have you]* often suspected that your spouse or partner has been unfaithful. Tell me about that. (What clues did you have? What did you do about it? Were you right?)	(7) has recurrent suspicions, without justification, regarding fidelity of spouse or sexual partner 3 = examples of unjustified suspicions with several partners or on several occasions with the same partner OR acknowledges trait he was screwing around with everyone	? (1) 2 3	73
	AT LEAST FOUR ITEMS ARE CODED "3"	(1) 3 → **PARANOID PERSONALITY DISORDER**	74

? = inadequate information 1 = absent or false 2 = subthreshold 3 = threshold or true

SCHIZOTYPAL PERSONALITY DISORDER

Note: Behavior should NOT be considered characteristic of Schizotypal Personality Disorder if it occurs exclusively during the course of Schizophrenia, a Mood Disorder With Psychotic Features, another Psychotic Disorder, or a Pervasive Developmental Disorder.

SCHIZOTYPAL PERSONALITY DISORDER CRITERIA

A pervasive pattern of social and interpersonal deficits marked by acute discomfort with, and reduced capacity for, close relationships as well as by cognitive or perceptual distortions and eccentricities of behavior, beginning by early adulthood and present in a variety of contexts, as indicated by five (or more) of the following:

49. You've said that when you are out in public and see people talking *[When you are out in public and see people talking, do]* you often feel that they are talking about you.

Tell me more about this.

(1) ideas of reference (excluding delusions of reference) ? (1) 2 3 75

3 = several examples

People notice me because I'm good-looking and I dress stylishly

50. You've said that you *[Do you]* often get the feeling that things that have no special meaning to most people are really meant to give you a message.

Tell me more about this.

51. You've said that when you are around people, you *[When you are around people, do you]* often get the feeling that you are being watched or stared at.

Tell me more about this.

? = inadequate information 1 = absent or false 2 = subthreshold 3 = threshold or true

52. You've said that you have *[Have you ever]* felt that you could make things happen just by making a wish or thinking about them.

Tell me about that.

(How did it affect you?)

(2) odd beliefs or magical thinking that influences behavior and is inconsistent with subcultural norms (e.g., superstitiousness, belief in clairvoyance, telepathy, or "sixth sense"; in children and adolescents, bizarre fantasies or preoccupations)

3 = several examples of such phenomena that influenced behavior and are inconsistent with subcultural norms

? 1 2 3 76

53. You've said that you have *[Have you]* had personal experiences with the supernatural.

Tell me about that.

(How did it affect you?)

54. You've said that you *[Do you]* believe that you have a "sixth sense" that allows you to know and predict things that others can't.

Tell me about that.

(How does it affect you?)

55. You've said that it often seems *[Does it often seem]* that objects or shadows are really people or animals or that noises are actually people's voices.

Give me some examples.

(Were you drinking or taking drugs at the time?)

(3) unusual perceptual experiences, including bodily illusions

3 = several examples of unusual perceptual experiences not due to drugs or a general medical condition

? 1 2 3 77

? = inadequate information 1 = absent or false 2 = subthreshold 3 = threshold or true

56. You've said that you have *[Have you]* had the sense that some person or force is around you, even though you cannot see anyone.

Tell me more about that.

(Were you drinking or taking drugs at the time?)

57. You've said that you *[Do you]* often see auras or energy fields around people.

Tell me more about that.

(Were you drinking or taking drugs at the time?)

OBSERVED DURING INTERVIEW	(4) odd thinking and speech (e.g., vague, circumstantial, metaphorical, over-elaborate, or stereotyped)	? (1) 2 3	78
CODE "3" IF ANY OF PARANOID CRITERIA (1), (2), (3), (4), OR (7) ARE CODED "3"	(5) suspiciousness or paranoid ideation	? (1) 3	79
OBSERVED DURING INTERVIEW	(6) inappropriate or constricted affect	? (1) 2 3	80
OBSERVED DURING INTERVIEW	(7) behavior or appearance that is odd, eccentric, or peculiar	? (1) 2 3	81
58. You've said that there are *[Are there]* very few people that you're really close to outside of your immediate family. How many close friends do you have?	(8) lack of close friends or confidants other than first-degree relatives 3 = no close friends (other than first-degree relatives)	? 1 2 3	82

? = inadequate information 1 = absent or false 2 = subthreshold 3 = threshold or true

59. You've said that *[Do]* you often feel nervous when you are with other people. What are you nervous about? (Are you still anxious even after you've known them for awhile?)	(9) excessive social anxiety that does not diminish with familiarity and tends to be associated with paranoid fears rather than negative judgments about self 3 = acknowledges excessive anxiety related to suspiciousness about other people's motives	? 1 2 3	83
	AT LEAST FIVE ITEMS ARE CODED "3"	1 3 ↓ **SCHIZOTYPAL PERSONALITY DISORDER**	84

? = inadequate information 1 = absent or false 2 = subthreshold 3 = threshold or true

SCHIZOID PERSONALITY DISORDER	SCHIZOID PERSONALITY DISORDER CRITERIA		
Note: Behavior should NOT be considered characteristic of Schizoid Personality Disorder if it occurs exclusively during the course of Schizophrenia, a Mood Disorder With Psychotic Features, another Psychotic Disorder, or a Pervasive Developmental Disorder or is due to the direct physiological effects of a general medical condition.	A pervasive pattern of detachment from social relationships and a restricted range of expression of emotions in interpersonal settings, beginning by early adulthood and present in a variety of contexts, as indicated by four (or more) of the following:		
60. You've said that it is *[Is it]* NOT important to you whether you have any close relationships. Tell me more about that. (What about your family?)	(1) neither desires nor enjoys close relationships, including being part of a family 3 = acknowledges trait	? 1 2 3	85
61. You've said that you would *[Would you]* almost always rather do things alone than with other people. (Is that true both at work and during your free time?)	(2) almost always chooses solitary activities 3 = acknowledges trait	? 1 2 3	86
62. You've said that you could *[Could you]* be content without ever being sexually involved with anyone. Tell me more about that. (Have you always had little interest in having sex?)	(3) has little, if any, interest in having sexual experiences with another person 3 = acknowledges trait	? 1 2 3	87

? = inadequate information 1 = absent or false 2 = subthreshold 3 = threshold or true

63. You've said that there are *[Are there]* really very few things that give you pleasure. Tell me about that. (What about physical things like eating a good meal or having sex?)	(4) takes pleasure in few, if any, activities [Note: Absence of pleasure especially applies to sensory, bodily, and interpersonal experiences.] 3 = acknowledges trait	? 1 2 3	88
ALREADY CODED ON ITEM (8) FOR SCHIZOTYPAL PERSONALITY DISORDER	(5) lacks close friends or confidants other than first-degree relatives	? (1) 2 3	89
64. You've said that it doesn't *[Does it NOT]* matter to you what people think of you. How do you feel when people praise you or criticize you?	(6) appears indifferent to the praise or criticism of others 3 = claims indifference to praise or criticism	? 1 2 3	90
65. You've said that *[Do]* you find that nothing makes you very happy or very sad. Tell me more about that. (ALSO CONSIDER BEHAVIOR DURING INTERVIEW)	(7) shows emotional coldness, detachment, or flattened affectivity 3 = occurring not exclusively during a Mood Disorder	? 1 2 3	91
	AT LEAST FOUR ITEMS ARE CODED "3"	(1) 3 ↓ **SCHIZOID PERSONALITY DISORDER**	92

? = inadequate information 1 = absent or false 2 = subthreshold 3 = threshold or true

HISTRIONIC PERSONALITY DISORDER	HISTRIONIC PERSONALITY DISORDER CRITERIA		
	A pervasive pattern of excessive emotionality and attention seeking, beginning by early adulthood and present in a variety of contexts, as indicated by five (or more) of the following:		
66. You've said that *[Do]* you like to be the center of attention. How do you feel when you're not?	(1) is uncomfortable in situations in which he or she is not the center of attention 3 = feels uncomfortable when not the center of attention	? 1 2 3 I'm a performer— I need to be on stage	93
67. You've said that *[Do]* you flirt a lot. Has anyone complained about this? (ALSO CONSIDER BEHAVIOR DURING INTERVIEW)	(2) interaction with others is often characterized by inappropriate sexually seductive or provocative behavior 3 = acknowledges complaints, describes inappropriate behavior, or observed to be inappropriately seductive	? 1 2 3 from interview observation (also says all his lovers have been upset by this)	94
68. You've said that you *[Do you]* often find yourself "coming on" to people. Tell me about it. (ALSO CONSIDER BEHAVIOR DURING INTERVIEW)			
OBSERVED DURING INTERVIEW	(3) displays rapidly shifting and shallow expression of emotions	? 1 2 3	95

? = inadequate information 1 = absent or false 2 = subthreshold 3 = threshold or true

69. You've said that you *[Do you]* try to draw attention to yourself by the way you dress or look. How do you do that? Do you do that all the time?	(4) consistently uses physical appearance to draw attention to self 3 = gives example and acknowledges that behavior occurs all the time	? 1 2 3 It's my style (also observation)	96
OBSERVED DURING INTERVIEW	(5) has a style of speech that is excessively impressionistic and lacking in detail	? 1 2 3 observed	97
70. You've said that you *[Do you]* often make a point of being dramatic and colorful. Tell me about that. (ALSO CONSIDER BEHAVIOR DURING INTERVIEW) (Do you like to show your emotions—for example, hugging people even if you don't know them very well or crying very easily?)	(6) shows self-dramatization, theatricality, and exaggerated expression of emotion 3 = acknowledges trait and at least one example my style—I'm not dull—I'm exciting—I let my feelings show	? 1 2 3	98
71. You've said that you *[Do you]* often change your mind about things depending on the people you're with or what you have just read or seen on TV. Tell me more about that.	(7) is suggestible (i.e., easily influenced by others or circumstances) 3 = acknowledges trait and at least one example	? 1 2 3	99
72. You've said that you *[Do you]* have lots of friends that you are very close to. How many? Who are they?	(8) considers relationships to be more intimate than they actually are 3 = claims to have many more "close" relationships than is believable	? 1 2 3	100
	AT LEAST FIVE ITEMS ARE CODED "3"	1 3 ↓ **HISTRIONIC PERSONALITY DISORDER**	101

? = inadequate information 1 = absent or false 2 = subthreshold 3 = threshold or true

NARCISSISTIC PERSONALITY DISORDER	NARCISSISTIC PERSONALITY DISORDER CRITERIA		
	A pervasive pattern of grandiosity (in fantasy or behavior), need for admiration, and lack of empathy, beginning by early adulthood and present in a variety of contexts, as indicated by five (or more) of the following:		
(73.) You've said that *[Do]* people often fail to appreciate your very special talents or accomplishments. Give me an example.	(1) has a grandiose sense of self-importance (e.g., exaggerates achievements and talents, expects to be recognized as superior without commensurate achievements)	? 1 2 (3) someday I'll have my own fan club	102
(74.) You've said that people have *[Have people]* told you that you have too high an opinion of yourself. Give me some examples of this.	3 = at least one example of grandiosity		
(75.) You've said that *[Do]* you think a lot about the power, fame, or recognition that will be yours someday. Tell me more about this. (How much time do you spend thinking about these things?)	(2) is preoccupied with fantasies of unlimited success, power, brilliance, beauty, or ideal love 3 = much of time spent daydreaming or in pursuit of unrealistic goals often daydreams about being a big star	? 1 2 (3)	103
76. You've said that *[Do]* you think a lot about the perfect romance that will be yours someday. Tell me more about this. (How much time do you spend thinking about this?)			

? = inadequate information 1 = absent or false 2 = subthreshold 3 = threshold or true

77. You've said that when you have a problem *[When you have a problem, do]* you almost always insist on seeing the top person. Give me some examples. (Why do you have to see the top person?) 78. You've said that *[Do]* you feel it is important to spend time with people who are special or influential. Why is that?	(3) believes that he or she is "special" and unique and can only be understood by, or should associate with, other special or high-status people (or institutions) 3 = acknowledges trait and at least one example *"Someone special to understand my problem"*	? 1 2 3 [3 circled]	104
79. You've said that it is *[Is it]* very important to you that people pay attention to you or admire you in some way. Tell me more about this.	(4) requires excessive admiration 3 = acknowledges trait and at least one example *I need for people to recognize my talent*	? 1 2 3 [3 circled]	105
80. You've said that *[Do]* you think that it's not necessary to follow certain rules or social conventions when they get in your way. Give me some examples. Why do you feel that way? 81. You've said that *[Do]* you feel that you are the kind of person who deserves special treatment. Tell me more about this.	(5) has a sense of entitlement (i.e., unreasonable expectations of especially favorable treatment or automatic compliance with his or her expectations) 3 = several examples *– wants free treatment* *– artists shouldn't have to bother about little rules*	? 1 2 3 [3 circled]	106
82. You've said that *[Do]* you often find it necessary to step on a few toes to get what you want. Tell me some instances of that. (Does that happen often?)	(6) is interpersonally exploitative (i.e., takes advantage of others to achieve his or her own ends) 3 = several examples in which another person is exploited	? 1 2 3 [1 circled]	107

? = inadequate information 1 = absent or false 2 = subthreshold 3 = threshold or true

83. You've said that *[Do]* you often have to put your needs above other people's.

Give me some examples of when that happens.

They should recognize that I'm a talented person

84. You've said that *[Do]* you often expect other people to do what you ask without question because of who you are.

(Does this happen often?)

85. You've said that you're *[Are you]* NOT really interested in other people's problems or feelings.

Tell me about that.

(7) lacks empathy: is unwilling to recognize or identify with the feelings and needs of others

3 = acknowledges trait OR several examples

? (1) 2 3 108

86. You've said that people have *[Have people]* complained to you that you don't listen to them or care about their feelings.

Tell me about that.

87. You've said that you are *[Are you]* often envious of others.

Tell me about it. (How often do you feel that way?)

(8) is often envious of others or believes that others are envious of him or her

I envy the big stars

3 = acknowledges trait and at least one example

? 1 2 (3) 109

88. You've said that *[Do]* you feel that others are often envious of you.

What do they envy about you?

Most people envy my good looks, my style

? = inadequate information 1 = absent or false 2 = subthreshold 3 = threshold or true

89. You've said that you *[Do you]* find that there are very few people that are worth your time and attention. Tell me about that. (ALSO CONSIDER BEHAVIOR DURING INTERVIEW)	(9) shows arrogant, haughty behaviors or attitudes 3 = acknowledges trait or observed during interview	? 1 2 (3) Observed during interview	110
	AT LEAST FIVE ITEMS ARE CODED "3"	1 (3) ↓ **NARCISSISTIC PERSONALITY DISORDER**	111

? = inadequate information 1 = absent or false 2 = subthreshold 3 = threshold or true

BORDERLINE PERSONALITY DISORDER	BORDERLINE PERSONALITY DISORDER CRITERIA		
	A pervasive pattern of instability of interpersonal relationships, self-image, and affects and marked impulsivity, beginning by early adulthood and present in a variety of contexts, as indicated by five (or more) of the following:		
90. You've said that you have *[Have you]* often become frantic when you thought that someone you really cared about was going to leave you. What have you done? (Have you threatened or pleaded with him/her?)	(1) frantic efforts to avoid real or imagined abandonment (**Note:** Do not include suicidal or self-mutilating behavior covered in item (5).) 3 = several examples happens whenever a relationship is ending— repeatedly calling ex-lover	? 1 2 3	112
91. You've said that *[Do]* your relationships with people you really care about have lots of extreme ups and downs. Tell me about them. (Were there times when you thought they were everything you wanted and other times when you thought they were terrible? How many relationships were like this?)	(2) a pattern of unstable and intense interpersonal relationships characterized by alternating between extremes of idealization and devaluation 3 = either one prolonged relationship or several briefer relationships in which the alternating pattern occurs at least twice	? 1 2 3 always had stormy relationships	113

? = inadequate information 1 = absent or false 2 = subthreshold 3 = threshold or true

92. You've said that you have *[Have you]* all of a sudden changed your sense of who you are and where you are headed.

Give me some examples of this.

93. You've said that your sense of who you are often changes *[Does your sense of who you are often change]* dramatically.

Tell me more about that.

94. You've said that you are *[Are you]* different with different people or in different situations so that you sometimes don't know who you really are.

Give me some examples of this. (Do you feel this way a lot?)

95. You've said that there have been *[Have there been]* lots of sudden changes in your goals, career plans, religious beliefs, and so on.

Tell me more about that.

(3) identity disturbance: markedly and persistently unstable self-image or sense of self

[Note: Do not include normal adolescent uncertainty.]

3 = acknowledges trait

? 1 2 3 (1 circled) 114

96. (circled) You've said that you've *[Have you]* often done things impulsively.

What kinds of things?

(How about . . .
. ✓. buying things you really couldn't afford?
. ✓. having sex with people you hardly know, or "unsafe sex"?
. ✓. drinking too much or taking drugs?
. . . driving recklessly?

(4) impulsivity in at least two areas that are potentially self-damaging (e.g., spending, sex, substance abuse, reckless driving, binge eating). (**Note:** Do not include suicidal or self-mutilating behavior covered in item (5).)

3 = several examples indicating a pattern of impulsive behavior (not necessarily limited to examples given above)

? 1 2 3 (3 circled) 115

always in credit card debt — drinking + drugging — sex

IF YES TO ANY OF ABOVE: Tell me about that. How often does it happen? What kinds of problems has it caused?

97. You've said that you have *[Have you]* tried to hurt or kill yourself or threatened to do so. 98. You've said that you have *[Have you ever]* cut, burned, or scratched yourself on purpose. Tell me about that.	(5) recurrent suicidal behavior, gestures, or threats, or self-mutilating behavior 3 = two or more events (when not in a Major Depressive Episode)	? 1 2 3 (2 circled) only once	116
99. You've said that *[Do]* you have a lot of sudden mood changes. Tell me about that. (How long do your "bad" moods last? How often do these mood changes happen? How suddenly do your moods change?)	(6) affective instability due to a marked reactivity of mood (e.g., intense episodic dysphoria, irritability, or anxiety usually lasting a few hours and only rarely more than a few days) 3 = acknowledges trait	? 1 2 3 (3 circled) always extremely moody	117
100. You've said that *[Do]* you often feel empty inside. Tell me more about this.	(7) chronic feelings of emptiness 3 = acknowledges trait	? 1 2 3 (1 circled)	118
101. You've said that *[Do]* you often have temper outbursts or get so angry that you lose control. Tell me about this.	(8) inappropriate, intense anger or difficulty controlling anger (e.g., frequent displays of temper, constant anger, recurrent physical fights) 3 = acknowledges trait and at least one example	? 1 2 3 (1 circled)	119

? = inadequate information 1 = absent or false 2 = subthreshold 3 = threshold or true

102. You've said that *[Do]* you hit people or throw things when you get angry.

Tell me about this.

(Does this happen often?)

103. You've said that *[Do]* even little things get you very angry.

When does this happen?

(Does this happen often?)

104. You've said that when you are under a lot of stress, you *[When you are under a lot of stress, do you]* get suspicious of other people or feel especially spaced out.

Tell me about that.

(9) transient, stress-related paranoid ideation or severe dissociative symptoms

3 = several examples that do not occur exclusively during a Psychotic Disorder or a Mood Disorder With Psychotic Features

? (1) 2 3 — 120

AT LEAST FIVE ITEMS ARE CODED "3"

(1) 3 — 121

↓

BORDERLINE PERSONALITY DISORDER

? = inadequate information **1 = absent or false** **2 = subthreshold** **3 = threshold or true**

ANTISOCIAL PERSONALITY DISORDER	ANTISOCIAL PERSONALITY DISORDER CRITERIA		
Note: Behavior should NOT be considered characteristic of Antisocial Personality Disorder if it occurs exclusively during the course of Schizophrenia or a Manic Episode.	B. The individual is at least age 18 years. C. There is evidence of Conduct Disorder with onset before age 15 years [as evidenced by at least two of the following:]	? 1 2 3 (3 circled)	122
105. You've said that before you were 15, you would *[Before you were 15, would you]* bully or threaten other kids. Tell me about that.	(1) (Before the age of 15) often bullied, threatened, or intimidated others	? 1 2 3	123
106. You've said that before you were 15, you would *[Before you were 15, would you]* start fights. How often?	(2) (Before the age of 15) often initiated physical fights	? 1 2 3	124
107. You've said that before you were 15, you hurt or threatened someone *[Before you were 15, did you hurt or threaten someone]* with a weapon, like a bat, brick, broken bottle, knife, or gun. Tell me about that.	(3) (Before the age of 15) used a weapon that can cause serious physical harm to others (e.g., a bat, brick, broken bottle, knife, gun)	? 1 2 3	125
108. You've said that before you were 15, you deliberately tortured someone or caused someone physical pain and suffering. *[Before you were 15, did you deliberately torture someone or cause someone physical pain and suffering?]* What did you do?	(4) (Before the age of 15) was physically cruel to people	? 1 2 3	126

? = inadequate information 1 = absent or false 2 = subthreshold 3 = threshold or true

109. You've said that before you were 15 you tortured or hurt animals on purpose. *[Before you were 15, did you torture or hurt animals on purpose?]* What did you do?	(5) (Before the age of 15) was physically cruel to animals	? 1 2 3	127
110. You've said that before you were 15, you robbed, mugged, or forcibly took *[Before you were 15, did you rob, mug, or forcibly take]* something from someone by threatening him or her. Tell me about that.	(6) (Before the age of 15) stole while confronting a victim (e.g., mugging, purse snatching, extortion, armed robbery)	? 1 2 3	128
111. You've said that before you were 15, you forced someone *[Before you were 15, did you force someone]* to have sex with you, to get undressed in front of you, or to touch you sexually. Tell me about it.	(7) (Before the age of 15) forced someone into sexual activity	? 1 2 3	129
112. You've said that before you were 15 you *[Before you were 15, did you]* set fires. Tell me about that.	(8) (Before the age of 15) deliberately engaged in fire setting with the intention of causing serious damage	? 1 2 3	130
113. You've said that before you were 15, you deliberately destroyed *[Before you were 15, did you deliberately destroy]* things that weren't yours. What did you do?	(9) (Before the age of 15) deliberately destroyed others' property (other than by fire setting)	? 1 2 3	131
114. You've said that before you were 15, you broke *[Before you were 15, did you break]* into houses, other buildings, or cars. Tell me about that.	(10) (Before the age of 15) broke into someone else's house, building, or car	? 1 2 3	132

? = inadequate information **1 = absent or false** **2 = subthreshold** **3 = threshold or true**

115. You've said that before you were 15, you lied a lot or "conned" *[Before you were 15, did you lie a lot or "con"]* other people. What would you lie about?	(11) (Before the age of 15) often lied to obtain goods or favors or to avoid obligations (i.e., "cons" others)	? 1 2 3	133
116. You've said that before you were 15, you sometimes stole or shoplifted things or forged someone's signature. *[Before you were 15, did you sometimes steal or shoplift things or forge someone's signature?]* Tell me about it.	(12) (Before the age of 15) stole items of nontrivial value without confronting a victim (e.g., shoplifting, stealing but without breaking and entering, forgery)	? 1 2 3	134
117. You've said that before you were 15, you ran away from home and stayed *[Before you were 15, did you run away and stay]* away overnight. Was that more than once? (With whom were you living at the time?)	(13) (Before the age of 15) ran away from home overnight at least twice while living in parental or parental surrogate home (or once without returning for a lengthy period)	? 1 2 3	135
118. You've said that before you were 13, you would *[Before you were 13, did you]* often stay out very late, long after the time you were supposed to be home. How often?	(14) (Before the age of 13) often stayed out at night despite parental prohibitions	? 1 2 3	136

? = inadequate information   1 = absent or false   2 = subthreshold   3 = threshold or true

119. You've said that before you were 13, you often skipped *[Before you were 13, did you often skip]* school. How often?	(15) (Before the age of 13) often truant from school	? 1 2 3	137
	AT LEAST TWO ITEMS ARE CODED "3" (i.e., "some" evidence of Conduct Disorder)	1 3	138

CRITERION C OF ANTISOCIAL PERSONALITY DISORDER MET; CONTINUE ON NEXT PAGE

GO TO PERSONALITY DISORDER NOT OTHERWISE SPECIFIED, PAGE 41

? = inadequate information 1 = absent or false 2 = subthreshold 3 = threshold or true

Question	Criterion	Rating	Item
Now, since you were 15. . .	A. There is a pervasive pattern of disregard for and violation of the rights of others occurring since age 15 years, as indicated by three (or more) of the following:		
Have you done things that are against the law—even if you weren't caught—like stealing, using or selling drugs, writing bad checks, or having sex for money? IF NO: Have you ever been arrested for anything?	(1) failure to conform to social norms with respect to lawful behaviors as indicated by repeatedly performing acts that are grounds for arrest 3 = several examples	? 1 2 3	139
Do you often find that you have to lie to get what you want? (Have you ever used an alias or pretended you were someone else?) (Have you often "conned" others to get what you want?)	(2) deceitfulness, as indicated by repeated lying, use of aliases, or "conning" others for personal profit or pleasure 3 = several examples	? 1 2 3	140
Do you often do things on the spur of the moment without thinking about how it will affect you or other people? What kinds of things? Was there ever a time when you had no regular place to live? (For how long?)	(3) impulsivity or failure to plan ahead 3 = several examples	? 1 2 3	141

? = inadequate information 1 = absent or false 2 = subthreshold 3 = threshold or true

(Since you were 15) have you been in any fights? (How often?) Have you ever hit or thrown things at your spouse or partner? (How often?) Have you ever hit a child, yours or someone else's—so hard that he or she had bruises or had to stay in bed or see a doctor? Tell me about that. Have you physically threatened or hurt anyone else? Tell me about that. (How often?)	(4) irritability and aggressiveness, as indicated by repeated physical fights or assaults 3 = several examples	? 1 2 3	142
Did you ever drive a car when you were drunk or high? How many speeding tickets have you gotten or car accidents have you been in? Do you always use protection if you have sex with someone you don't know well? (Has anyone ever said that you allowed a child that you were taking care of to be in a dangerous situation?)	(5) reckless disregard for safety of self or others 3 = several examples	? 1 2 3	143

? = inadequate information **1 = absent or false** **2 = subthreshold** **3 = threshold or true**

How much of the time in the last 5 years were you not working? IF FOR A PROLONGED PERIOD: Why? (Was there work available?) When you were working, did you miss a lot of work? IF YES: Why? Did you ever walk off a job without having another one to go to? IF YES: How many times did this happen? Have you ever owed people money and not paid them back? (How often?) What about not paying child support, or not giving money to children or someone else who depended on you?	(6) consistent irresponsibility, as indicated by repeated failure to sustain consistent work behavior or honor financial obligations 3 = several examples	? 1 2 3	144
IF THERE IS EVIDENCE OF ANTISOCIAL ACTS AND IT IS UNCLEAR WHETHER THERE IS ANY REMORSE: How do you feel about [LIST ANTISOCIAL ACTS]? (Do you think what you did was wrong in any way?)	(7) lacks remorse, as indicated by being indifferent to or rationalizing having hurt, mistreated, or stolen from another 3 = lacks remorse about several antisocial acts	? 1 2 3	145

? = inadequate information 1 = absent or false 2 = subthreshold 3 = threshold or true

AT LEAST THREE ITEMS ARE CODED "3" — 1 3 — 146

CRITERION A OF ANTISOCIAL PERSONALITY DISORDER MET

CRITERIA A, B, AND C ARE CODED "3" — 1 3 — 147

ANTISOCIAL PERSONALITY DISORDER

? = inadequate information 1 = absent or false 2 = subthreshold 3 = threshold or true

PERSONALITY DISORDER NOT OTHERWISE SPECIFIED

This category is for disorders of personality functioning that do not meet criteria for any specific personality disorder. An example is the presence of features of more than one specific personality disorder that do not meet the full criteria for any one personality disorder ("mixed personality") but that together cause clinically significant distress or impairment in one or more important areas of functioning (e.g., social or occupational). This category can also be used when the clinician judges that a specific personality disorder that is not included in the classification (e.g., self-defeating personality disorder) is appropriate.

(1) 3 → 148

PERSONALITY DISORDER NOT OTHERWISE SPECIFIED